A Fireside Book

Published by Simon & Schuster

New York

London

Toronto

Sydney

Singapore

walking

yoga

Incorporate Yoga Principles into
Dynamic Walking Routines
for Physical Health, Mental Peace,
and Spiritual Enrichment

ila sarley and garrett sarley

FIRESIDE
Rockefeller Center
1230 Avenue of the Americas
New York, New York 10020

FIRESIDE and colophon are registered trademarks
of Simon & Schuster Inc.

For information about special discounts for bulk purchases,
please contact Simon & Schuster Special Sales:
1-800-456-6798 or business@simonandschuster.com

Designed by Chris Welch
Photographs © 2002 by Cynthia Del Conte
Illustrations © 2002 by Katherine Jones

Manufactured in the United States of America

10 9 8 7 6 5 4 3 2 1

Library of Congress Cataloging-in-Publication Data is available.

ISBN 0-7434-2197-3

acknowledgments

We'd like to thank:

Our family members, friends, and mentors who have helped us on our path, especially Ken Anbender, who gave us language to describe yoga in life and whose loving counsel helped us through a very difficult time. Elizabeth Lesser and Stephan Rechtschaffen, co-founders of the Omega Institute, for their friendship, support, and generosity of spirit. Ling Lucas, our book agent who gave us great advice, cheered us on, and encouraged us to express ourselves through this medium. Tracy Behar and Brenda Copeland, our editors at Pocket Books. Stephanie Gunning and Grace Welker for their administrative and editorial support. Katherine Jones for her line drawings. Cynthia Del Conte, our photographer. Catherine Simprini for her experience, advice and feedback. Ramona Anne Kelly for critiquing the manuscript and for her artistic and creative support during our photo shoots.

This book is dedicated:

To our parents, James and Mary Jane Kelly and Bud Sarley and Jean Green. You taught us to pursue truth and integrity and encouraged us to follow our own individual heart's calling. We have truly been blessed.

To our teachers Swami Kripalvanandaji and Yogi Amrit Desai who lovingly inspired and guided our yoga practice, giving us the opportunity to dedicate our lives to the eternal and life-changing experience of yoga.

contents

walking
yoga

introduction

Inevitably, the idea for this book was born on a walk.

It was one of those magical fall days in the northeastern woods; the trees were a firestorm of color, the sun a warmhearted friend, and the air like tonic for the lungs. In stark contrast to the beauty of the day, though, was the internal state in which we found ourselves. It was the end of a long and stressful week, and we both woke up that Saturday morning with the feeling that all was not well with the world; somehow life was to be feared rather than embraced.

We also felt out of sorts with each other. Disconnected.

Do you know the feeling when you look at your partner and he or she seems more like an enemy than a friend? Well, that's how we felt: out of sorts with each other, the world, and ourselves.

Two hours later we found ourselves talking, laughing, filled with energy and a renewed sense of confidence and well-being. Such a radical change in two hours!

What was the therapy that produced such profound results? Could we bottle it? Could we count on it?

We had spent those two hours doing our yoga practice and walking through the woods at a state park near our house—simple activities really. When we reflected on our experience that October morning, we realized that we had been practicing the spirit of yoga during our walk as well as while doing our yoga postures. Our hatha yoga practice flowed into a walking yoga practice. The combination of the two was a potent antidote to the stress and depression we were experiencing that Saturday morning. If walking yoga could affect us this way, we reasoned, it could affect others just as powerfully.

Walking yoga gives you a direct experience of the body as well as access to the body's natural intelligence and its ability to generate robust health and spiritual well-being. In order to practice walking yoga on streets and trails, you need to first practice yoga on the mat. The postures and breathing techniques you will learn in this book will give you a solid foundation for developing a daily yoga practice in which you gain a degree of mastery not only within your body but also within your mind. Nothing can take away the struggles that life presents, but having a regular walking yoga practice can strengthen you physically and mentally, giving you a foundation for handling whatever comes at you. Yoga done on the mat and yoga done on a walk offers you access to a deep reservoir of calm, balance, and strength, even in the midst of an emotional storm.

We both discovered yoga in our late teens and moved into the same yoga ashram, dedicating our lives to studying the depth and breadth of this remarkable ancient science. For the last twenty-seven years, yoga has captivated our hearts and minds and has functioned as a guiding light for our personal and spiritual development, as well as our relationships to each other, our work, our family, and our community. Our yoga practice has grounded us in both the good times and the bad, and in this book we offer you some of the insights, practices, and tools we have used to keep our lives balanced and whole.

We hope that you find the practice of walking yoga as rich as we do. We have tried many forms of physical and spiritual exercise and, in our opinion, the practice of yoga and walking together is the gentlest, least injurious, most nurturing, deeply satisfying, and delightful way to generate total health. We have studied with yoga masters, priests, and shamans; traveled to sacred pilgrimage sites around the world; run marathons; climbed mountains; fasted; and dedicated a lifetime to the practice of yoga and meditation. But in the end it is the simple pleasure of a walk in the woods and the exquisite nourishment of a gentle yoga practice that keep us deeply connected to our bodies and souls.

walking yoga

If you ask people what motivates them to exercise, you'll find a common theme that changes as we age. We exercise in our twenties and thirties to look good, in our forties and fifties to improve our health, and in our sixties and seventies for longevity. You don't usually hear people say they exercise for spiritual enrichment; most of us find our solace and nourishment for the soul in a church, mosque, temple, or synagogue. The wonderful thing about the practice of walking yoga is that you get all the benefits of exercise—looking good, improving your health, life extension—in addition to the deeper benefits of nourishing your spirit. When you incorporate the unifying elements of yoga while walking, it's not just good for the body; perhaps most important, walking yoga is good for the soul. Benefits such as increased confidence, peace of mind, and insight are less tangible but no less important than the physical benefits of exercise.

The synthesis of walking and yoga happens in the moment when you are fully present: when you walk in time with the rhythm of the breath and your sensory awareness is so acute that you actually tingle with the electricity of life. We call this type of walking, walking yoga, in which every step generates more energy and power in the body, creativity in the mind, and connection to spirit.

Walking yoga is about nurturing your body and soul, not about forcing yourself to work out because you should. It is a form of exercise that—done properly—reliably produces an experience of coming home to yourself. As you develop your walking yoga practice, it becomes a flow of meditative movement and one-pointed focus that allows you to tap into a powerful, mystical space inside you. Gaining access to this inner space gives you a sense of confidence, strength, and balance. You automatically begin to look better and feel better about yourself and your life.

With walking yoga, we have developed an active practice that will help reduce stress and produce peace of mind for those of you who can't imagine sitting still to pray or meditate. In walking yoga, the aim is to be present and focused on the sensations of the movement you are making. You employ rhythmic breathing and sensory awareness to help the mind concentrate on the task at hand. In a way similar to what's done in a sitting meditation practice, in walking yoga you bring the mind, which often wanders, back to the present moment and experience.

The inspiration for a dynamic practice that is good for the body *and* the spirit is not new. Just look at religious and spiritual movements such as Sufis whirling (sacred dance) and Christian mystics walking the labyrinth (walking meditation) to find examples of active prayer, in which the body is engaged while praying to the Almighty. World religious traditions—East, West, and indigenous—all contain some form of physical discipline as a way to higher spiritual states, whether the practice be one of diet, posture, walking, fasting, breathing, singing, or the laying on of hands.

Walking, however, has been the preferred form of meditation practiced by some of the greatest thinkers of modern times. Søren Kierkegaard, Charles Darwin, and Friedrich Nietzsche all considered walking an essential part of their health and genius. Henry David Thoreau and Ralph Waldo Emerson used walking as a form of meditation and were some of the first Westerners to integrate yoga philosophy into their walking practice.

Even today, those devoted to a spiritual life use walking in their practice; Buddhists include walking meditation as a core practice in their contemplative life; Jesuits build ambulatories for walking prayer; Hindu monks walk on their spiritual pilgrimage to holy sites; and Australian aborigines take "walkabouts," primarily to find themselves in relation to the world of nature and spirit. Walking seems to lend itself to freeing the mind, opening the heart, and connecting us to a higher spirit.

Most forms of contemplative walking incorporate the discipline of quieting the mind and focusing on the present moment through breath and sensory awareness. Walking meditation can be a potent portal to the here and now. What makes walking yoga unique is that it takes this basic practice to a deeper level by engaging the body's rhythms and natural intelligence, which the practice of yoga helps you attune to, to generate integration and health in the body, mind, and spirit. In addition to stilling the mind and being present, you listen for the natural evolutionary urges that occur through a tuned and healthy physical system. In essence you become a more powerful receiver for the natural intelligence that is in and around you.

The Benefits of Yoga

Yoga is a philosophy as well as a physical practice. The word *yoga* means "union," and the true aim of yoga is to connect us with our deeper integrated self. This practice begins by developing an awareness of being in your body. An increase in body awareness manifests in an increase in the vital energy or life force (see page 22) of your body, mind, and spirit, leading you to a healthier way of being. Yoga has three primary definitions: skillfulness in action, equilibrium, and absorption. Each definition sheds light on how to generate the central experience yoga promises, the experience of union with the self.

Skillfulness in Action: Yoga teaches that in each moment there is a way we can act that is perfectly in line with the natural life force. Athletes talk about skillfulness in action as being in the "zone," where things seem to slow down, the basket appears bigger or the balance beam feels a foot wider. We know we have achieved this skillfulness when our actions seem to flow spontaneously, effortlessly, and automatically. Skillful action is about being fully engaged in life in such a way that it becomes the natural expression of yourself acting in accordance with the universal life force. When you act skillfully you find that not only do you create a seamless inner experience but you also become more effective and powerful.

Skillful action is an integration of the two basic pulls in nature: inertia and growth. We are simultaneously being pulled to accept ourselves the way we are and also to grow and change. When you focus too much on the former, you become static and lazy. Focus too much on the latter, and you wear yourself out with striving and wind up damaging your body or mind. Either extreme robs you of peace, energy, and health.

In yoga, we practice skillfulness in action by developing a sense of mastery in the postures, continually improving and growing into the discipline while respecting the natural boundaries and limitations of the body at any given time.

Equilibrium: Equilibrium is the practice of experiencing life just as it is, without running from it or trying to squeeze more out of it. It is about finding and knowing your center no matter what life brings you. When you engender equilibrium, you are firmly connected to your center and can respond with balance and comfort to life's changing circumstances.

Most of the time we resist the feelings and sensations that naturally arise from events, reacting rather than responding to them. Consequently, when we are called to grow and change, to challenge our preexisting mental belief systems, or when our expectations are not met, we experience turbulence of some kind. Learning to negotiate turbulence and to ride the waves of mental and emotional upset frees you to accept life as it comes and to allow change to occur naturally and automatically.

For example, every time you stretch in a yoga posture, you generate sensations that are turbulent and at times uncomfortable. You practice equilibrium by fully accepting your experience. An easy way to translate accepting your experience is simply to observe the sensations occurring in your body, then relax into the stretch, even if it is uncomfortable. Within three to four deep breaths, the sensations in your body will move from discomfort to comfort. Practicing equilibrium during yoga postures acts as a metaphor for life. Pain and pleasure are two sides of the same coin, and the practice of equilibrium gives you the perspective to embrace both fully.

Absorption: When you can contain turbulence, you create the conditions for the last definition of yoga: absorption. When you drop into pure experience without trying to influence it, you become absorbed in the moment. And when you become absorbed in the moment, you can experience yourself as you are. Through absorption you find that you start to touch a part of yourself that is eternal and sustaining. You begin to experience the self that is already complete and at peace.

In yoga, absorption is not so much a practice as a result. When you practice skillfulness in action and equilibrium in both life and yoga, the result is being absorbed in the present moment.

Experiencing the integrative power of yoga rests on building a strong foundation on a physical level. Mental, emotional, and spiritual balance are enhanced when your body is healthy and working smoothly. A regular practice of hatha yoga and breathing exercises improves the functioning of all the major systems in the body.

THE SKELETAL SYSTEM

The framework of the body, the bones, increases in strength through use. Many of the standing and balancing poses of yoga are weight-bearing exercises, which help to keep the bones healthy and strong. In addition, yoga postures move the joints and, with practice, slowly increase their range of movement. Limited range of movement causes stiffness in the joints. You've probably heard the expression "use it or lose it." Nowhere is this more applicable than in the joints and the skeleton.

The spine is central to the health of the body and affects and is affected by every movement your body makes. The arms, legs, and chest are all attached to the spine via the shoulder girdle, ribs, and pelvis. So if the arms and legs don't have full range of motion, the spine must compensate by extra bending and twisting. By contrast, if the spine is not functioning properly, the arms, legs, and head can't move freely either. The movement principles of hatha yoga keep the spine elongated and flexible by creating space between the vertebrae, allowing blood and fluids to bathe them, then compressing fluids out of the vertebrae. This process is particularly helpful for the intervertebral disks, which have no blood supply of their own and are dependent on sponge action to keep their thick pads of cartilage healthy. As we age, we develop poor posture and lose our youthful flexibility. This loss causes the disks to become thin, brittle, and easily injured. There is a saying, "You are as young as your spine is flexible." Hatha yoga is a reliable regimen for keeping the spine healthy and every joint loose and free.

THE MUSCULAR SYSTEM

Healthy and efficient muscles that are long, relaxed, and toned, combined with well-conditioned fascia, bring the spine and skeleton into an appropriate relationship with one's center of gravity. The fascia are the connective tissue that hold together and compartmentalize the bundles of fibers that make up muscle tissue and allow easy movement of one muscle or muscle group relative to another. Yoga postures cleanse the muscles and fascia of accumulated stress hormones through deep stretching and increased circulation. A regular practice of standing and floor postures will keep the muscles and fascia strong and flexible.

THE CIRCULATORY SYSTEM

The blood traveling through the circulatory system carries nutrients, oxygen, antibodies, and hormones to the cells of the body. It also removes waste products from the cells. Hatha yoga postures increase the flow of blood to all parts of the body, helping to flush toxins from the organs and muscles.

THE LYMPHATIC SYSTEM

The lymphatic system is a network of lymphatic vessels and lymph nodes (or storage sacs) that extends to almost all parts of the body. Yoga massages and stimulates the draining of the lymphatic system, promoting the appropriate transportation of infection-fighting white blood cells and the waste products of cellular activity throughout the body.

THE NERVOUS SYSTEM

The central nervous system consists of the brain and the spinal cord. It controls the sensations and movements of all the parts of the body and influences thoughts, emotions, and memories. The autonomic nervous system includes the involuntary systems of the body and works through two sets of nerves, the sympathetic and the parasympathetic. This system is directly related to stress and your response to it. Through the practice of yoga, the heartbeat slows, respiration becomes deeper and slower, blood pressure lowers, and you activate the relaxation response, relieving stressed nerves. In addition, physical pressure on the nerves is relieved by keeping the spine and joints flexible and the muscles relaxed and supple.

From a spiritual point of view, a strong nervous system allows you to increase your nervous system's capacity to carry energy. You may have heard of the seven chakras, or energy centers in the body (see page 137). Chakras are made up of bundles of nerves in different parts of the body, where energy can be either generated or blocked. Yoga postures work directly on these nerve bundles to enhance energy production and remove blocks.

THE DIGESTIVE SYSTEM

The digestive system produces fuel for the body, and yoga can help increase its efficiency and effectiveness. Almost every yoga posture positively affects the digestive organs. When you assume a posture and add breath to the pose, you will find that you create a gentle yet powerful massage for your abdominal organs and muscles, which helps to stimulate the digestive system and promote assimilation. Many poses also stimulate the eliminative function, cleansing the intestinal tract, the kidneys, liver, and skin, to produce a healthy, youthful glow.

THE RESPIRATORY SYSTEM

The respiratory system provides oxygen to and eliminates carbon dioxide from the body. The breathing exercises used in yoga help to clean the lungs' air sacs and increase the lung's capacity to take in and absorb oxygen. The deep breathing employed in the postures assists in the elimination of toxins carried from the cells by the bloodstream to the lungs for exhalation as carbon dioxide. Increased energy and mental alertness are the results of a healthy respiratory system. Because yogis believe that spiritual energy is carried into the body on the wings of the breath, a strong respiratory system is essential for a deeper walking yoga practice.

THE ENDOCRINE SYSTEM

Endocrine glands regulate most of the body's functions through chemical substances called hormones and neurotransmitters. You'll no doubt notice a feeling of well-being after practicing hatha yoga. This sensation is a direct result of the toning and detoxification of the endocrine system. Specific postures help strengthen and balance glandular function; for example, the Forward Bends massage the organs in the neuroendocrine glands (pituitary, hypothalamus, thyroid, and adrenals), helping to balance hormonal flow. The Shoulder Stand and Headstand rejuvenate the thyroid gland and pineal gland respectively.

The Benefits of Walking

A walking routine is easy to get into. No matter what age you are, what shape you are in, or where you live, most likely you can walk. Walking is free and doesn't require any type of special equipment. Although we recommend investing in a pair of good walking shoes, we've seen sherpas (guides) in Nepal walking up steep mountains with enormous packs on their backs in sandals.

Walking is a great way to maintain overall physical health and is recommended as one of the most beneficial remedies to stress. Since our lives can be overwhelming and stressful, we need to do something on a regular basis to counteract the negative results of stress. At the very least, stress creates discomfort and has a detrimental effect on our health. When our bodies are overstressed, we feel anxious, isolated, and irritable. We sleep less well, and our digestion is off.

Modern psychological research shows the correlation between certain physical and biochemical states and stressful reactions. When a person experiences stress, the brain responds by releasing a variety of chemicals, such as adrenaline and cortisol, into the bloodstream to combat the stress and stay in control. This is called the fight or flight response and gives a momentary energy boost to do whatever needs to be done to survive. The muscles tense, the heart beats faster, breathing and perspiration increase, the eyes dilate, and the stomach may clench. If the cause of stress is not discontinued, the body will secrete more hormones that increase blood sugar levels to sustain energy and raise blood pressure. If we don't manage the stress in our lives, we overtax our endocrine system, exhausting the glands that produce the hormones that help us resist disease. The American Medical Association has stated that stress is the cause of 80 to 85 percent of all human illness and disease, making it the number-one cause of death in humans.

Walking on a regular basis helps to cleanse the body of its accumulated stress hormones and leads to more vibrant health. Research has shown that neurotransmitters such as endorphins, which have a positive effect on the human body, are released from the pituitary gland during vigorous exercise. Scottish and British scientists have identified the endorphin molecule and noted its association with the feeling of euphoria and well-being, particularly after exercise. When we regularly engage in aerobic exercise (see page 126), our immune systems perform better, we sleep more deeply, and we digest our food more completely. The combination of yoga and walking is a tonic for the negative side effects of stress and depression, and is as powerful as any mood-altering food or drug on the market.

Regular walking, at least three times per week for a sustained period of 30 minutes or more, helps reestablish total physical health because it engages so many of the vital systems of the body. Specifically, walking

- Strengthens the heart, increasing the flow of blood and oxygen throughout the body
- Increases muscular coordination, improving strength, flexibility, and stamina
- Promotes weight loss (if done for a minimum of 20 minutes, and preferably 30 minutes, at least three times per week, during which you increase your heart rate to the point of breaking a sweat)
- Encourages better posture
- Reduces levels of unhealthy stress hormones
- Improves digestion
- Relaxes and calms the mind

Walking is also good for the bones. Because physical activity makes bones stronger and denser, exercise is essential in building healthy bones and warding off osteoporosis, a bone-weakening condition that affects more than 28 million Americans, 80 percent of them female. "Physical activity, through its load-bearing effect on the skeleton, is likely the single most important influence on bone density and architecture," concludes the 1996 U.S. Surgeon General's Report on Physical Activity and Health. Weight-bearing exercise is defined as any activity you do on your feet that works your bones and muscles against gravity. Walking is one of the best forms of weight-bearing exercise because it is enjoyable, it is easy to commit to, and the likelihood of injury is extremely low.

When done vigorously enough to increase your heart rate to an aerobic level several times a week, walking can also provide the amount of aerobic exercise the body requires. Since the only aspect of health that yoga doesn't fully stimulate is the cardiovascular development associated with aerobic exercise, combining walking with yoga is especially important for those of you who are already yoga practitioners.

Combining the age-old activity of walking with yoga—skillfulness in action, equilibrium, and absorption—allows you to create an ideal physical and spiritual practice, one that permits you to meditate while you move. The spiritual dimension of life is intimately connected to the physical. Without this direct experience of being alive in the body on a regular basis, we forfeit the essence of spirituality—being truly alive.

More often than not, we disconnect physical exercise from our hearts and spirits; as a result regular, consistent practice becomes a promise we rarely keep. Instead, we relate to exercise as something we should do but never find the time for, a further hardship that we avoid. Our failure to exercise becomes a source of guilt and tension, adding pressure to our already overcommitted lives. But when you approach exercise from an integrated place, you actually start to crave the good feelings that are generated. The discipline needed to practice comes naturally and effortlessly.

Nurturing Body and Soul

Sarah's Story

Sarah is a student of ours who was overweight and struggling with a lack of confidence and low-level depression. She came from a family of athletes, and even though she tried to keep up with the runners in her family, she never really enjoyed the exercise and she kept injuring herself. Since exercise and physical condition were highly valued in her family, being overweight and out of shape made her feel like a failure and diminished her self-esteem. For Sarah, exercise had become a way to gain acceptance from her family and friends, but she got no pleasure out of it.

Her family and friends all recommended exercise to help Sarah with both her weight and her depression, but no matter how hard she tried she could never stick to a regular workout. Sarah came to our walking yoga workshop as a skeptic. Her mother had given it to her as a gift for her thirty-eighth birthday. She was injured from her latest try at a kickboxing class and was the heaviest she had been in years.

Yoga's emphasis on listening to your inner needs and inclinations gave Sarah a way to find pleasure in the exercise she was doing. The good feelings built on themselves, and before we knew it, Sarah was practicing walking yoga for thirty minutes every morning. Now that she was able to change her re-

continued on next page

lationship to exercise to one in which nurturing and loving her body was primary, she could sustain a regular practice.

Does Sarah sound like someone you know, or does she have echoes within your own experience? Have you gotten into some form of sports or exercise only to give it up because of injury or in reaction to constantly pushing yourself? The key to health and longevity is to pick activities that generate a natural physical and spiritual attunement by creating a sense of wholeness, connection, and integration.

We all tend to find excuses for not taking time for our exercise practice. "It's too cold outside." "I'm too tired." "I'm starving." "The kids need my attention." "I have too much to do around the house." You quickly convince yourself that you'll feel better if you clean the house or get dinner ready and, since you are so hungry, you have some snacks while you clean, cook, and connect with your family. By nine o'clock you're stuffed with food that you never really enjoyed and, yes, you have accomplished a few more chores, but if you really think about it you are no closer to being complete with your chores than when you started. Chores tend to multiply without ceasing.

At some point you have to realize that if you don't do something that nurtures your body and mind regularly, you will feel stressed out and depressed all the time. If you don't take care of yourself, you can be certain you'll end up feeling like your life has no meaning and your to-do list is infinite. You can eventually find yourself in a very negative state of being, taking your unhappiness out on those closest to you. No matter how legitimate your excuses for not exercising are, in the end you are the one who suffers, because you feel unfulfilled.

Ila writes of her experience with overcoming resistance to taking time for herself: "I walk in the door after a long day at the office, promising I'll take time to do something good for myself. There are dishes in the sink, mail and magazines all over the dining room table, and clothes on the floor in the living room and bedroom. I feel pulled to start cleaning and get dinner ready, and I crave something sweet.

"Somehow, instead of diving into cookies and chores, I manage to walk up the hill behind my house, my mind focused on unfinished conversations, stuff to do at work, and knotty problems still unresolved. For the first ten minutes of my walk I hardly notice where I am because my thinking is so intense, but then I remember my practice. I bring my awareness to my breath, then the movements of my body, the sensations of the air, the sounds, the sights, and the quiet stillness around me. Suddenly, what is going on inside my head seems loud and insignificant. My awareness becomes more focused and my head begins to clear. It is that time just before sunset when everything slows down and prepares for the night to close in. I consciously unwind in tune with nature's flow.

"There is a tall, old, and elegant oak tree along the road that I walk. The tree seems so complete in its being. Branches fully extended to absorb the sun's rays, its whole life is dedicated to the one pursuit of absorbing nutrients to grow. The simplicity of its existence is a sharp contrast to the complexity of my life. I draw a deep breath in as I walk, and the fresh, simple pleasure of being in nature thoroughly rejuvenates me. I am grateful I broke away from the constant activity of my life to get a new perspective.

"Now I'm inspired, so when I come back into the house I ignore all the work waiting to be done and I take another fifteen minutes to relax, breathe, and do my yoga stretches. By the time I'm finished, I feel better about the dishes in the sink, I take time to cook a nourishing meal, and I have energy to tackle my to-do list, which doesn't seem so endless anymore."

At the beginning of your walking yoga practice, before you have developed a routine you naturally look forward to, it is vital just to get yourself moving. Drag yourself away from the endless list of to-dos, put your sneakers on, and head out and practice walking yoga, even if you can take only fifteen minutes. Tell yourself that you only have to walk for five minutes. Just get started, and you'll be amazed how good you feel, and how quickly. Usually the good feeling builds and you'll want to keep walking.

In this book we will explore walking in different modes to show how bringing awareness to each of these forms creates the experience of yoga—connection with the self, others, life, and spirit. Sometimes we need to be alone, other times to have company; sometimes we need to walk fast, other times to walk slowly. Within walking yoga there are natural seasons for different types of walking, just as there are natural rhythms to our changing needs. The first important point is to notice your natural rhythms, and ask yourself, What do I need today? The second point is to practice the type of walking you need in such a way that it is truly yoga. When your walk becomes an extension of your yoga practice, it becomes a reliable path for mental peace, physical health, and spiritual enrichment.

Walking yoga is one of the best ways to get out of your head and into your spirit—opening your eyes to a much bigger world outside yourself, the mystical world of the sacred. Walking yoga means bringing presence and awareness to your walking so that your body becomes your temple and place of sanctuary. The practice of walking yoga uplifts the spirit, calms the mind, and nurtures the soul. It is the perfect antidote to the high-stress, fast-paced lives many of us live. You don't want your daily form of exercise and rejuvenation to pressure you as much as your busy life. You want a practice that can nurture you body and soul, and walking yoga is that practice.

Chapter 2

understanding yoga

Thousands of years ago in India, inquiry into metaphysical matters occupied a preeminent place in the culture. Spiritual attainment was highly respected and rewarded, and the brightest minds focused on understanding the deeper questions of being human. Questions such as What is the nature of happiness and unhappiness? How do our actions affect our sense of inner peacefulness? Who am I? What does it mean to have an inner life? What does personal growth look and feel like? This focus on the inner life produced the science of yoga—as applicable now as it was six thousand years ago.

One of the cornerstones of science is the ability to produce predictable results. If you're in New York City and you want a cup of tea, you get your teapot off the shelf, fill it with water, and turn on the stove. Several minutes later the water starts to bubble and then boil. If you measure the temperature of the water, you'll find it boils at 212 degrees Fahrenheit (at sea level). If you are in London and the urge for tea strikes, you'll find the water also boils at 212 degrees Fahrenheit though, being in London, you might measure it at 100 degrees Celsius. Because you can perform this experiment over and over and get the same results, you can say that the temperature at which water boils is scientifically proven.

Another principle of science is that you don't have to hold a particular belief in order for it to work. Water boils at 212 degrees whether you are a Catholic, a Muslim, a Jew, or an atheist. You may be skeptical about water boiling at 212 degrees, or you may fervently believe this to be the case, yet, you will find your skepticism or faith has no impact on the water's boiling point.

The science of yoga is the same: It produces predictable results and is unaffected by our belief systems. What, then, did the ancient yogis discover in their scientific approach to inner life? Essentially, that our desire for happiness, spirituality, inner peace, and connection with others depends not on the outer circumstances of our lives but on the level of vital life force energy available to us on the inside.

Vital Life Force Energy

What do we mean when we say life force or vital energy? Think of a healthy, vibrant plant. The leaves are green and shiny, the stem and branches are strong and lifted to the sky, and both the leaf and root structures are lavishly developed to take in the optimal amount of sun, water, and nutrients. The plant is filled with life force and radiates vitality. Likewise, when we are filled with life force and vital energy, we feel happy, peaceful, spiritual, and connected.

When we lack this life force, we are more like a wilting plant with faded leaves. When we are depleted of life force and vital energy, we feel unhealthy, insecure, anxious, and isolated. Most of our lifestyle choices and responses to life's challenges end up depleting more vital energy than they generate. We often function like buckets with holes. The water (life force energy) runs out faster than it comes in, and gradually the level of water diminishes. Unfortunately, as the water level lowers, we age more quickly. When the bucket empties, we die. When you start to make choices that generate more energy than they consume, you begin to retard the aging process.

On a pilgrimage to India in 1990, we met a Jain monk who followed a yogic tradition of complete renunciation; he owned no material possessions, ate food only when it was offered by the local townsfolk, and spent his days studying yogic scripture, teaching, and meditating. What was amazing about this man was his energy and charisma. He was full of vital energy and radiated strength, intelligence, and dignity. His chosen lifestyle generated such life force and vitality that he seemed dressed in the garments of a king, despite his humble trappings. This simple monk, who owned nothing but his own conviction and intelligence, illustrates how the science of yoga works.

Yoga has lasted for centuries because it outlines practical, reliable, scientific steps to achieve its results. These steps work whether you understand them or not, whether you practice them in America or England, and whether you can touch your toes or haven't seen them in a couple of years. It doesn't matter whether you are rich or poor, married or single, famous or unknown, you are responsible for the maintenance of your own inner life force.

The key to maintaining a vital inner life force lies in mastering our responses to life, not trying to master what happens to us. No one ever really controls us or decides what to do except us. People may lie to, hurt, steal from, or cheat us, but we decide how we will react, and these choices ultimately create our reality.

Creating Our Reality

There were once twin brothers who grew up to lead very different lives. One had all the things we dream about, a

continued on next page

loving and stable marriage, healthy and vibrant children, a well-paying job, and the respect of the community where he lived. He was active in drug- and alcohol-abuse prevention programs in local schools and spent spare time and money volunteering to support children, like himself, who had lost parents to early deaths.

The other brother had all manner of problems. He seemed to go from relationship to relationship, often attracting women who were abusive to him or whom he abused. If he had success at a job, he would somehow sabotage himself, and his success would be short-lived. He had two children by different women but couldn't develop rapport with either of them and seldom saw them. He developed a dependence on alcohol and lived a lonely and dispirited existence.

When both brothers were contacted as part of an identical twin research program, they were asked the following question: What event in your past do you consider most powerful in making your life come out the way it has? Amazingly enough, both brothers gave the same answer. "The death of my father from alcoholism when I was ten." Identical twins, identical event early in life, even identical impact of the event, yet vastly different responses. This is the starting point of yoga; each of us has the power to make our life a positive experience or a negative one.

If you have the power to make your life a more positive experience, how do you use that power? What do you do on a practical, everyday level? The answer lies in understanding that every action either consumes more vital energy than it generates or generates more energy than it consumes. That is, every action we perform either enhances our vitality or depletes it. In a profound way, any action that enhances our vitality can be classified as a form of yoga practice.

For example, if you are a coffee drinker, you may notice that when you drink a cup of coffee in the morning to get you going, you get a temporary boost in energy only to feel low in energy later in the morning. After giving your body an initial lift, caffeine can create a wired, nervous feeling, even causing the hands to tremble. When we measure the total effect of drinking coffee, we find that for many people it actually consumes more energy than it generates. Worse still, the body becomes dependent on these doses of caffeine, and regular coffee drinkers go through caffeine withdrawal when deprived of coffee for a couple of days, often developing headaches and restless sleep patterns.

THE PHYSICAL BODY: FROM DEPLETION TO VITALITY

Stan, a friend of ours, was forty-five pounds overweight, smoked pot and drank beer in the evenings, ate a diet rich in fats and sugars, got little exercise, and spent most of his time working or watching television. Although he was only forty-seven, he looked close to sixty. He had large, dark circles under his dull eyes, his skin had a papery and dried out look to it, he had arthritis in his hands, and he moved like an old man. People who met him were always surprised to learn his age. When his brother was diagnosed with colon cancer, the shock and fear forced Stan to take a good look at himself in the mirror. Stan decided to change his lifestyle. He gave up eating sugar and began a strict low-fat diet. He started to practice meditation and walking yoga nearly every day. He adjusted his work schedule to accommodate these more nurturing habits and learned to become more efficient and less stressed over work deadlines. He also cut back significantly on smoking pot and drinking.

In two months Stan looked like a different person. It was astounding to see. The circles under his eyes were almost gone, and his skin was shiny and healthy. Stan lost twenty pounds, his eyes were bright, his arthritis improved and, he noticed, his memory was sharper too. Beyond the obvious physical effects, he reported that he was enjoying life more than he ever had. He looked and felt ten years younger than he had with his old lifestyle.

THE MENTAL AND EMOTIONAL BODIES: FROM DEPLETION TO VITALITY

Ancient yogis also discovered that energy is generated and expended not only on a physical level but on a mental and emotional level, and that there is an interactive relationship between the physical and the mental and emotional. Modern medicine is now confirming what the yogis knew long ago. Numerous studies have shown that when we are mentally or emotionally stressed, our arteries constrict, our heart rate increases, and our digestion is less efficient. In addition, research conducted by members of the medical community interested in holistic medicine, including Dr. Dean Ornish's work at the Preventive Medicine Research Institute in Sausalito, California, has shown that the heart and immune system are strongly affected by the degree to which we love and are loved. Physical actions such as walking, meditation, and yoga postures are coming to be recognized as effective treatments for depression and anxiety and are regularly being prescribed to help people manage stress and stay positive and happy. In his book *The Aerobics Program for Total Well-Being*. Dr. Kenneth Cooper writes, "Many physicians believe that exercise is nature's best physiological tranquilizer. In addition to using exercise as a means of controlling depression, psychiatrists are using it as a way of relieving some types of stress and emotional anxiety."

When you take care of yourself by living a healthy, balanced life, your vitality increases dramatically. Do you remember a time when you successfully committed to exercising regularly or eating a moderate, balanced diet? Remember how great you felt, not just physically but mentally too? This is because these activities increased your vital energy, which then directly affected your mental and emotional health. When your body and mind are healthy and filled with life force, your skin looks shiny and has a healthy glow, your posture is straight and tall, and both your body and your mind develop to take in the optimal amount of nutrition and information to stimulate growth. You radiate vitality and passion for life.

Integrating Vital Energy

Vital life force energy is the product of our being integrated in body, mind, and spirit. We thrive when all parts of our life are integrated and connected. We lose this sense of integration when we do not listen to all the parts of ourselves, for example, when we decide to eat another portion even though our stomach is full, because the mind is bored or distracted. Sometimes, the mind insists on doing something that is ostensibly good for us, such as starting an exercise program. However, gaining vital energy is not a matter of forcing yourself to start a walking regime, a hatha yoga practice, or a healthy diet. A vital lifestyle always incorporates some measure of self-discipline, but the discipline must come from a love of the activity and the results it produces.

Our friend Susan practiced yoga and meditation on a regular basis, ate a well-balanced diet, and appeared to love her work as a counselor, which she treated as a form of service. Susan was also a devoted parent and an active member of her community. For years Susan seemed to thrive on her busy lifestyle, content spending her time making her children, her husband, her clients, and her friends and neighbors the priority in her life.

But sometime around her thirty-ninth birthday, Susan started to dread going to work and had less interest in the social activities she used to love so much. She found herself tiring easily and catching colds and the flu with unexpected regularity. When she began to investigate her condition, she found that she had developed a case of chronic fatigue syndrome, characterized by an assembly of symptoms that can be summed up best as an overall lack of energy.

What Susan began to see was that part of her efforts to care for others was a sense of discomfort with taking time for herself. She had given all her attention and energy to being a mom, a wife, a helping professional, a spiritual seeker, and an active community member, and she was pretty much ignoring her own needs and desires. This disconnection eventually sapped her life force, even though she was practicing what looked like a yogic lifestyle. Susan eventually began to understand her need to have appropriate boundaries and to put self-nurturance higher on her priority list. Gradually, as she started to integrate her personal needs with the needs of others, she began to regain her vital energy, and her emotional, mental, and physical health improved.

Susan's story illustrates our inability to cheat the life force principle. A yoga teacher once said that no matter what you do, you can't deceive your own cells. Each of our cells faithfully records the effect of each of our actions, both gross physical actions and subtle mental and emotional actions. Your real inner experience is scribed in your biochemistry, and only you can know the truth of what is written there.

In essence, yoga is defined as those actions that produce thriving on a cellular and biochemical level as well as on less tangible mental, emotional, and spiritual levels. This is an important point because it puts the controls in your hands. You can actually do things that increase cellular health and overall vitality, and you can learn to be sensitive to your biochemical health. Yoga also challenges you to practice skillfulness in action because, like Susan, you will find that certain actions can cause vitality at one time in your life but not at others. You also find that what works for someone else may not work exactly the same way for you. It is not the action that makes it yoga but the effect produced. This means that each of us must approach the practice of yoga through our own experience, continually monitoring our vitality to test the impact of our actions.

Swami Kripalvanandaji, an accomplished yoga master who devoted his entire adult life to the practice of yoga, cautioned his students not to believe anything about yoga that they didn't directly experience themselves. Given this philosophy, the yoga practitioner is always reinterpreting the practices prescribed by yoga and making them more personal and more powerful in producing predictable results. The practicing yogi steers by what produces thriving and life force, not by a particular set of disciplines. The yogi monitors the effects, not just the actions.

Tuning In to the Body's Intelligence

The Greek philosopher and scientist Archimedes is famously quoted as saying, "Everything is intelligent!" What do we mean by saying something is intelligent? Consider the following: When a car encounters a wall, it must stop because it has no intelligence in it. When you add a driver to that car, he can drive around the wall because he has a destination in mind and the intelligence to interact with the wall. If the car and its driver come to a river, the driver can get out and build a bridge because he still has a specific destination in mind beyond the river. No matter how many obstacles the driver of the car encounters, he will interact with each obstacle in a creative way to further his efforts to reach his destination. In the end, the driver may even discard the car itself and walk in the direction of his destination.

The most fundamental way to define intelligence is as the ability to respond to changing circumstances with a particular end in mind. Nature provides a myriad of examples of how intelligence works. If a rock sits on top of a seed, the seed changes its natural tendency to grow straight up, sending out a longer shoot to run under the rock until it reaches the edge and grows straight up from there. Eventually, it may even get strong enough to push the rock aside. When a tree grows in the shade, it will always orient its growth toward the sun, even if it has to distort its whole trunk to do so. We have seen mighty pine trees grow out of the face of solid granite walls of stone, having found the only hospitable cracks in the walls to support their life. Clearly everything in nature is interacting with everything else with a particular goal: to sustain more life, and more life force.

Nature's Intelligence

We were standing on the top of a mountain just off the John Muir Trail in California's Sierra Nevada when we saw the principle of natural intelligence in grand relief. We were looking across the valley at a glacier, which had formed in a north-facing col of the Ritter range, one of the most rugged areas of the whole Sierra range. At the head of the glacier, there was no life, just cold rock and bright, sterile snow, etched sharply against the skyline in the afternoon sun. As our eyes followed the glacier downhill, we could see life emerge from that initial matrix of snow, sun, and stone.

At first the only evidence of life was reddish patches on the snow itself, where the sun had melted the snow and the resulting water formed a basis for a type of red algae to grow. Soon the water eroded enough of the rock to form sand and made the conditions just right for certain alpine plants to grow. As we looked even further downhill, we could see grasses appearing as the glacier gave way to a rushing stream. Insects could live in the grasses, small birds nested and thrived by eating the insects, and a family of marmots sheltered themselves in a boulder field, where they fed on the seed of the mountain grasses. At the bottom of the chasm was a lake, filled with fish and surrounded by forests, inhabited by deer, bear, mountain lions, small rodents, and many types of birds, insects, and reptiles.

We sat back in wonder at the obvious intelligence at work here: Within less than half a mile and six thousand feet in elevation, nature had created a rich and diverse ecosystem out of a sterile mix of ice, snow, rock, and sun! Nothing was wasted. Every material was used to create more life, and the more life there was, the more life was built onto it. The more life force there was in the system, the more life force was possible in the system.

LISTENING TO THE BODY'S INTELLIGENCE

The natural intelligence of nature is also active inside us. The easiest place to see the body's intelligence at work is in the digestive process.

When we eat food, we start one of the most mysterious and miraculous chemical processes imaginable. Our bodies are able to turn vegetables, grains, beans, oils, eggs, milk, fish, and meat into some of nature's most sophisticated and subtle chemical compounds. These same core chemicals are in all of us, whether a vegan living on sprouts and carrot juice in San Francisco or a Masai warrior subsisting on cow meat and blood on the Kenyan prairie.

In order to recognize whether something generates vitality or depletes it, we must learn to listen to the messages of the body and its ability to guide us from our own source of natural intelligence. These body messages are particularly important when our habits and addictions short-circuit our motivation and negatively affect our commitment to a certain energy-producing action. Yoga engages you in becoming more aware of your body and the state of its vital energy, and this is the first step toward generating more life force and vitality in the body.

Fortunately, the body communicates information about the state of your life force in a predictable progression of increasing volume, starting with intuition and moving through urge, discomfort, pain, chronic pain, and then disease.

Intuition

First, the body signals you with an intuition about something you need or a condition that should change. Often you don't really pay attention to this initial intuition because the message is faint, and you're too busy with life to take care of such subtle, seemingly insignificant messages. For example, one day while you are biting into some french fries a thought might pop into your head that maybe this is why you feel that pain in your side. Your intuition is telling you that you may be eating too much fried food.

Urge

When you ignore your intuition, the message becomes a little louder, and you feel the urge to change. You start telling yourself, "I really need to respond to this feeling. Fried food really isn't good for me. I should make a change." These thoughts begin to occur more and more frequently. Unfortunately, the power of your entrenched habits, security mechanisms, and comfort-producing patterns often make change difficult or scary, so you continue to ignore the urge. You may think to yourself, "I know fried foods are hard to digest, but I don't want to give up my favorite comfort foods. Besides, maybe it's something else and, to be honest, I have more important things to think about."

Discomfort

When you ignore your urges long enough, you start to experience the message about the state of your health as an occasional discomfort. Now you often think to yourself, "I've really got to make a change here. I can feel a pain in my side and I realize my digestion, sleep patterns, and feeling of health are worse." You notice the discomfort in your side when you drive a car and sometimes when you lie down, and you notice that the discomfort comes and goes. The discomfort is isolated to an area on the right side of your body, and you wonder if it is your gallbladder or liver. At this point you may acknowledge the dull awareness of the discomfort by taking mild over-the-counter medication, and you may consider seeing a doctor. Sometimes your distress over the discomfort leads you to *increasing* addictive patterns to drown out the sound of the coming storm. You focus on killing the messenger rather than listening to the message.

Pain

If you are successful in ignoring the discomfort, your body turns up the volume and the discomfort becomes actual pain. At this point you start to pay attention, but instead of looking for the causes in your lifestyle and emotional patterning, you start consuming stronger medication on a more regular basis. You schedule an appointment to see a doctor, and she confirms that you have a sluggish gallbladder and, if you are lucky, recommends a change in diet. Your reaction can range from praying that it will go away on its own to making a vow to change your diet. Often the challenge of cleaning up your diet is more difficult than you imagined, and you start to backslide into ignoring your condition.

Chronic Pain

Now the pain is amplified to a chronic pain. It hurts all the time and truly begins to affect your lifestyle. In this phase the slightest bit of stress on your system, such as the intake of any rich food or alcohol, will cause a flare-up in physical pain to the point where you become dysfunctional. If you don't immediately change your diet, you will risk having your gallbladder fail. At this time you begin to consider medical intervention.

Disease

From chronic pain, it is only a short hop to the state of disease, where the life force and health of your body are permanently damaged, at least to some degree. Eventually the disease becomes such a wound to the life force that the body can no longer sustain itself, and at this point severe medical intervention, such as surgery, is required. If you haven't responded to the messages your gallbladder has been sending you with a change in diet and exercise, then you are forced to have surgery to take care of the gallbladder's needs. At some point in this process, if the disease is not successfully reversed, death comes.

All health issues, both physical and mental, go through this progression, and the earlier you respond to the warning signals, the sooner you will return to wholeness. The good news is that through the practice of yoga you can become more sensitive to the quieter messages of intuition, urge, and discomfort, before they become the louder communications of pain, chronic pain, and disease.

Garrett's Story

"Twenty-five years ago, when I first became interested in yoga, my practice consisted of doing the basic postures and breathing exercises of hatha yoga. As my commitment deepened and my study expanded, I began to broaden my definition of yoga. I became convinced that a more accurate description of yoga was the practice of listening to my body's natural signals, and learning to distinguish natural signals from learned signals. As I practiced this broader interpretation I began to see improvements in my health and ultimately learned to use this practice to deal with any health challenges that presented themselves in my life.

"My genetic background was not strong, with early deaths on both sides of my family, and my early childhood nutrition was not geared to produce health. As a result, I grew up with a number of allergies and a recurrent case of asthma, as well as recurrent pain in my knees and in the backs of my legs. Amazingly, my asthma went away completely in the first year of my yoga practice. I remember clearly the exact time of its departure, never to return. I had been practicing deep relaxation at the end of my yoga sessions and was able to enter successively deeper states of stillness and ease. Finally, at the end of one class, I became so still that I relaxed at a core level, which I had never allowed myself to do before. I felt I was okay the way I

continued on next page

was, that I was not at risk in life, and that I could drop the inner psychic tension, which was the deep source of the asthma. I felt a psychic and physical weight lift off my chest. From that day forward I have not had another asthma attack."

Ultimately we've come to believe that for every choice you make you have to ask yourself, "Am I feeding my life force or not?" This is the fundamental question. When you focus your life on nurturing the life force within you, then every action you take is either productive or counter to that focus. Every response we have to life, to others, to our feelings, and to our spirit either enlivens us or deadens us. True health flows only from a gradual increase in the life force.

From a yogic perspective, the body's intelligence works on levels beyond maintenance through digestion of food, elimination of waste, and resistance to disease. In the same way that nature uses every material and organism as a basis for more life, the body's intelligence, when followed, propels us toward a higher level of functioning. When you do something that generates life force, you start to feel better. You also start to notice other ways you keep yourself from feeling even better, such as staying in an unfulfilling relationship, lying at work, or always saying yes to others. As you begin to discontinue those actions that deplete your life force, you move into a higher level of awareness.

When you incorporate a spiritual practice such as yoga into your life, your focus on the inner life generates greater sensitivity to the subtle experiences of the body. Your radar gets more sophisticated, and you start to learn what the life force feels like on a kinesthetic level. You begin to notice what being fully alive feels like. This is especially true with yoga postures because the postures and breathing techniques cause a tangible increase of vital life force energy, providing a powerful experience of feeling balanced and alive.

Chapter 3

yoga on the mat

In order to practice walking yoga on the trails and in the streets, you need to practice yoga on the mat as well. The popularity of yoga has spread in the United States because of the branch of yoga referred to as hatha yoga. When you or your friends attend a typical yoga class, you learn and practice the poses (or *asanas*, which is the Sanskrit word for postures or exercises) and breathing techniques of hatha yoga. Literally translated, *hatha* means "power" or "effort," which reflects the intention of controlling the body. The word can also be understood to mean "complementary forces," because *ha* translates into "sun," and *tha* into "moon."

Yoga postures are the perfect complement to a walking practice. On a physical level yoga tones, strengthens, and lengthens the musculature of the body; promotes ease of movement in the joints; and facilitates proper structural alignment. To get the most out of your walk, it's important that your muscles be both strong and flexible and that the relationship between the skeleton, muscles, and connective tissue be balanced and aligned. Yoga postures help your structural system function more harmoniously, which will help you avoid injury and sustain healthy walking. Practicing yoga will also enhance your walking stamina and endurance. As you increase your level of fitness, you'll find that your confidence and spirit are lifted, affecting your whole outlook on life. You'll feel taller, younger, and generally more comfortable in your body.

Flexibility is an important ally of walking. When you walk, you want your stride to be as uninhibited as possible and, when you walk regularly, your muscles tend to shorten and tighten up. Practicing yoga before and/or after your walk will strengthen muscles that are weak, stretch those that are tight, and condition the connective tissue, which can increase range of motion and help reduce the likelihood of injury. Muscular tension and imbalanced alignment can inhibit your natural walking gait and increase the likelihood of injury.

How do we get so stiff in the first place? Inflexibility in the musculature of the body is generated from our everyday activities, both physical and mental. For example, many of us spend a good portion of life sitting down. We sit in the car or train going to and from work, at desks through the workday, during meals, and while watching television. As a result, the hamstring muscles, back muscles, and neck muscles contract and shorten. Take a moment right now to stand up and bend forward with your arms dangling toward the floor and your head dropped forward. You'll probably notice that the muscles along the back of your body feel tight and painful, from your calves all the way up to the base of your skull.

Muscle stiffness also occurs when our everyday responsibilities and emotional reactions to life cause us stress. The body stores everything we have ever experienced just like the memory banks of a computer. Those experiences that we have not digested and completed get stored as tension in the musculature. Stressful reactions to things that happen cause the body to release powerful chemicals, such as adrenaline and cortisol, into the bloodstream. These chemicals lodge themselves in the muscles, causing them to stiffen up.

When muscles stay continually contracted, they shorten, become less supple, less strong, and less able to absorb the shock and stress of various types of movement. The support for the skeletal system is undermined, and strong muscles can be injured when compensating for weak ones. Excessive muscular tension evolves into a more complex physical imbalance because habitually tense muscles reduce the blood flow to the muscle cells. This reduction in blood flow results in a lack of fresh oxygen and essential nutrients being carried to the cells and prevention of toxic waste products being carried out of the cells. The system imbalance causes stiffness in the muscles and other related illnesses such as hypertension, high blood pressure, and sciatica. The practice of yoga postures counteracts the detrimental effects of stress and muscular tension and restores flexibility and mobility through the postures and breathing exercises.

Introduction to Walking Yoga Posture Practice

The best place to develop a formal yoga practice is in a regular class or at a workshop or retreat with a qualified teacher. There are yoga classes available in almost every town and city. Going to a yoga retreat is an especially good way to learn because you have the time for intensive practice, and you can learn at a deeper level. Because there are many details involved in doing a posture correctly, having the expertise of a good teacher is an invaluable aid. Having said that, we do include a routine of formal yoga postures with which you can begin.

When you practice hatha yoga, it's helpful to have a blanket, a six-foot-by-three-inch strap, and a yoga or sticky mat. Blankets can be used for support and comfort in certain postures and provide warmth under and over your body in final relaxation. A yoga strap will aid your ability to reach and stretch in specific postures, and a sticky mat gives you stability in standing postures. For more information about yoga supplies, you can call Hugger-Mugger at 800-473-4888 or visit their web site, www.huggermugger.com.

We most often practice our yoga postures in the morning after our walk, but yoga postures can be done anytime (except after a meal), and they will always provide the same benefit. We recommend practicing 30 minutes of hatha yoga every day and taking an hourlong yoga class at least once a week. You can practice your yoga postures before or after your walk, although if you are taking a strenuous hike, it is best to practice yoga before you walk. We find that practicing at the same time every day, whether it is in the morning or in the evening, helps you stay consistent.

Combining breath with the postures is as important in formal yoga as it is when walking. Chapter 4 includes instructions for complete yogic breathing and Ujjayi breathing (see pages 97 and 101). We always recommend both of these breathing techniques when combining breath with postures. In the beginning, focus on attaining the correct form of the posture. You can add breath as your practice develops.

Practice yoga postures on an empty stomach, and wear loose-fitting or stretch clothing. If you are pregnant and just beginning your yoga practice with this book, consult with a yoga teacher experienced in teaching pregnant women before starting. You are caring for two lives now, and some yoga postures should be modified or avoided during pregnancy. During menstruation, do not practice any yoga postures that constrict the abdomen or Kapalabhati breathing (see page 102). If you have a serious medical condition such as heart disease and have no experience with yoga, consult your doctor and take a yoga class to learn which postures to modify and which to avoid so you can assure complete safety as you practice. Be sure to inform your yoga teacher of your condition before starting your class.

READ THE INSTRUCTIONS FOR EACH POSTURE

The following sequence can be practiced by just about anyone, but you must read the instructions and notes before practicing to receive the maximum benefits of the postures and to avoid injury. When you begin a posture, become aware of the alignment of your head, neck, shoulders, spine, hips, knees, and feet. Misalignment puts too much strain on the movable parts of the body, making them prone to injury, particularly as we age. So start slowly and gently, and pay attention to the alignment of your body. Occasionally practicing in front of a mirror helps to check your alignment.

LISTEN TO YOUR BODY

Remember to apply the principle of skillfulness in action (see page 8) by continually improving and growing into the postures while at the same time respecting the natural boundaries and limitations of your body. If the stretch feels too intense, back off of it a little until you feel the sensation of the stretch without pain. In general, you want to be able to hold a posture for at least 30 seconds, and up to one minute. After you have developed strength through your practice, if you can't hold a posture for this amount of time it is usually because you are straining too much. Do not hold your breath while practicing yoga postures.

BE IN THE MOMENT

As you practice the postures, focus your awareness on exactly what you are doing in the moment. Next, coordinate your breath with your movement and sink into the sensations of the stretch rather than simply finishing it in order to go for your walk. In general, when the torso moves up and expands, inhale. When the torso moves down and bends forward, exhale. If possible, breathe through your nose and use Ujjayi breathing (see page 101).

SURRENDER TO THE EXPERIENCE

In yoga we learn to focus our attention in the present moment, which in yogic terms is referred to as absorption (see page 9). In order to experience absorption you must develop the capacity to be relaxed and comfortable in the present moment. That means whatever is going on, whether it be painful or pleasurable, you can remain present for it. In other words, when a stretch feels good you enjoy the pleasure of it, and when a stretch is uncomfortable you relax into that experience too. As odd as it sounds, when you relax into the intense and often uncomfortable sensation of stretching tight muscles, it becomes pleasurable.

PRACTICE SENSORY AWARENESS

The ability to experience the present moment starts with sensory awareness. You increase awareness in hatha yoga because the process of learning and practicing the postures involves concentration. Sensory awareness and concentration are developed by paying attention to the sound and flow of the breath as well as the sensations you experience as you move through each posture. Once you have moved into the correct form of the posture, hold the position. If you can relax at this stage, you will automatically move deeper into the stretch and experience a deep sense of relaxation.

Try this posture, called Yoga Mudra, to see what we mean. Sit on your heels with your legs bent under you. Rest your palms on your knees. Start the posture by focusing on your breath. Take long, deep breaths through the nose, feeling the sensation of air entering the tips of your nostrils. Notice the temperature and sensations of the air on your arms and hands.

Inhaling, slowly lift your arms straight out in front of you until they are in line with your shoulders, parallel to the floor. Move in slow motion, focusing on the feeling of your arms floating through the air and listening to the sound of your breath in the background. Exhaling, bring your arms back behind you so that you can interlace your fingers.

Interlace your fingers, straighten your arms, and roll your shoulders back and down. Move slowly enough that you can adjust to the stretch in the shoulders and down the arms. Take two long, deep breaths, and let the trapezius, deltoid, triceps, and biceps muscles relax, elongate, and stretch. Continue to listen to the sound of the breath, allowing the movement to become a meditation in motion.

Take a deep breath in and, as you exhale, fold forward, lowering your torso and head toward the floor and raising your arms behind you toward the ceiling as far as you can. Keep your elbows straight. Once in the full position, folded forward with your arms behind you in the air, use the breath to help you relax into the stretch. You may feel discomfort in the shoulders and biceps at first. This initial discomfort of stretching tight muscles will evolve into pleasure as you breathe into the sensation of the stretch. Hold the pose for 10 to 30 seconds.

Beginners: If sitting on your heels is uncomfortable, place one or two blankets between your thighs and calves or sit cross-legged on the floor. You may not be able to bend forward because of restriction in your shoulders or arms. If this is the case, simply sit up straight, lift your arms until they are engaged, and hold for 10 to 30 seconds. If you can bend forward but not far enough to get your forehead to the mat, you can place a pillow or blanket between your chest and your thighs and one on the mat directly under your forehead.

Two Approaches to Walking Yoga Posture Practice

MEDITATIVE MOVEMENT

The meditative movement approach to the postures is excellent when you've had a very stressful day, when you are tired and tense, or when you are not feeling well. Your priority is to nurture, heal, and relax your body and to counteract the effects of the day. With meditative movement, you move from one stage of a posture to the next as slowly as possible, as if you are in slow motion. You approach the postures as a form of meditation in motion.

To enhance this experience, keep your eyes open, and gaze softly at a point in front of you while you are in standing or balancing poses. Close your eyes when doing floor poses and when you pause in the standing postures. Closing your eyes facilitates drawing your attention inward to the sensations of your movements and the sound of the breath. As you develop, your yoga practice becomes a flow of meditative movement, rhythmic breathing, and one-pointed focus that allows you to tap into a mystical and nurturing space inside of you.

VIGOROUS YOGA FLOW

Practice the vigorous yoga flow approach when you've got a lot on your mind and can't seem to concentrate, or when you're feeling sluggish or sleepy and you want to challenge and strengthen your body and increase your energy. Flow through the posture sequence from one movement to the next, and once you are in the full pose hold the posture for at least 30 seconds. While you hold the posture, take long, deep breaths without a pause between the inhalation and the exhalation. In the vigorous flow, the pace of your movements is faster than in the meditative movement. We recommend starting with the Sun Salutation (see page 59) and repeating it 3 times, then continuing with standing postures before doing any floor poses.

Warming Up

We always start our posture sessions with movements designed to gently prepare the body for the deeper yoga stretches. When you warm up the body, you activate the sensory motor system, which communicates to the muscles to relax and elongate. Taking time to warm the body up will help prevent injury and make your postures much more enjoyable.

NECK ROLL

The slow and simple movements of the Neck Roll provide a great way to start your yoga session. Neck Rolls gently release tension in the neck and shoulders and alert your body and mind that your yoga practice is starting. Practicing Neck Rolls while doing complete yogic breathing (see page 97) with Ujjayi breathing (see page 101) calms and centers the body and mind.

How to do the pose:

1. Sit in a chair or find a comfortable seated position on the mat. Keep your spine straight, regardless of the sitting position you choose. If you are in a chair, keep both feet flat on the floor; if you are on your mat, sit in an easy cross-legged position. Close your eyes during this exercise to facilitate the quieting of your mind and relaxation of your body.

2. With your arms resting easily at your sides, rest your hands, palms facing upward, on your thighs. Inhale very slowly, lifting your shoulders to your earlobes. Exhaling, lower them slowly back down. Repeat three times.

3. Take a deep breath in using the Ujjayi breath (see page 101), and as you exhale bend your head forward, dropping your chin toward your chest. Keep your spine upright and shoulders relaxed. Now let the head roll all the way around, in a big circle. You can imagine that you have a pencil pointing straight out of the top of your head like

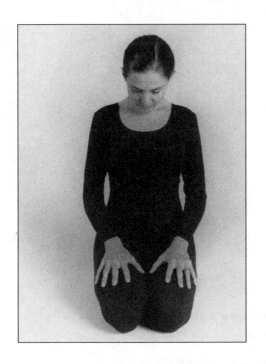

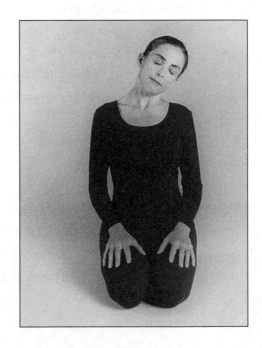

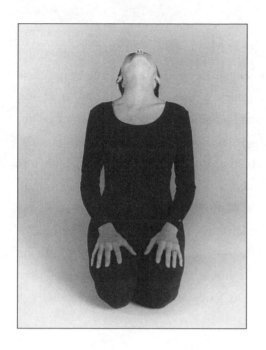

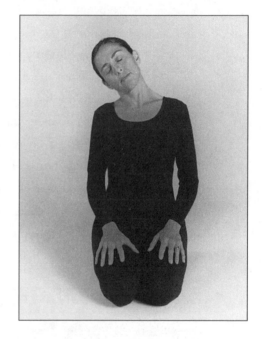

an extension of your spine, and you are drawing big circles on the ceiling. Try to move slowly, in time with the breath, dropping your chin to the chest on the exhalations and rolling around and toward the back with the inhalations.

4. Roll your head clockwise 3 times and counterclockwise 3 times, keeping your face, abdomen, and hands soft and relaxed as you move. Move in slow motion, with each rotation timed to correspond with one full inhalation and exhalation.

5. Bring your head back into an upright position and sit still for three more breaths.

BUTTERFLY

In this position, the legs look like the wings of a butterfly at rest. The Butterfly pose opens the hip joints, helps relieve arthritis of the knee, hip, and pelvic joints, and increases blood flow to the abdomen, pelvis, and lower back.

The Butterfly can be a challenging hip-opening pose. To get the most from the posture and avoid injury, move into the pose slowly, allow your knees to remain as high as they need to be, and avoid the urge to bounce your knees toward the mat. When first trying the Butterfly, focus on relaxing and stretching your groin muscles, not on bringing your knees to the mat. If you cannot grab your feet with your hands, or to help your spine elongate, you can also place a bolster or pillow under each knee for added support.

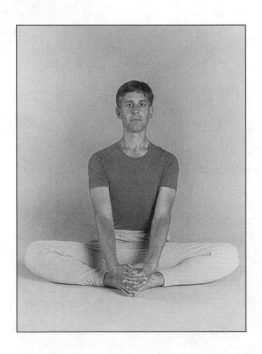

● ● ●

How to do the pose:

1. Sit on the mat with your legs out in front of you. Bend your right leg, and with your hands draw the heel of your right foot in toward your groin. Do the same with your left leg, placing the soles of your feet so they are flat against each other. Clasp your feet near your toes with both hands and draw your heels slowly toward your groin. Bring them in as close as is comfortable.

2. Lift your torso, straighten your back, and extend your spine upward while continuing to clasp your feet with your hands. Open your chest by pressing your shoulders back, bringing your chin parallel to the floor, lengthening the back of your neck, and looking forward.

3. Pressing your thighs firmly into the mat, press your knees away from your torso and down toward the mat.

4. Take several long, deep breaths and close your eyes. Relax into the stretch.

SUPINE LEG STRETCH

The Supine Leg Stretch is done with the help of a yoga strap, scarf, or soft belt. This posture is wonderful for opening the hip joints and increases flexibility in the spine, the whole pelvic region, and the leg muscles, while increasing blood circulation to the legs. It makes stretching tight hamstrings and calf muscles safe and enjoyable.

How to do the pose:

1. Lay on your back on the mat with your legs together and your feet flexed so that they are flat as if they were pressed against a wall. Bend your right leg and wrap a yoga strap or belt on top of the ball

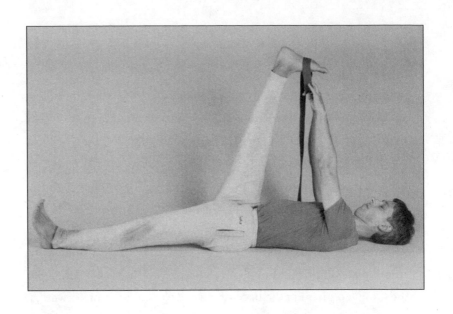

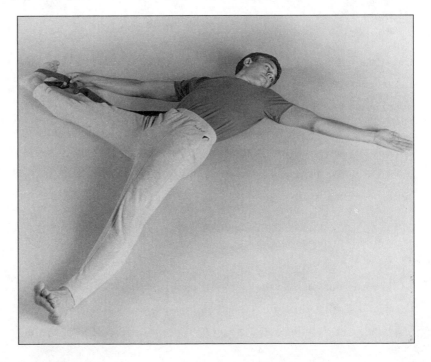

walking yoga

of your right foot. Wrap the ends of the belt around your hands so that your arms are extended straight out from your shoulders and your hands are as close to your feet as possible.

2. Straighten and extend your right leg toward the ceiling. It is important to keep the left leg straight and pressed down into the floor; keep your left leg engaged by contracting the muscles of your front thigh and lifting your kneecap. Press the back of your knee toward your mat.

3. As you lift your right leg, you might find that at a certain point it starts to bend. Stop at that point to work the posture with your leg straight and your foot flexed. Pressing the heel of your right leg toward the ceiling and the toes down toward your head will accentuate the stretch in the back of your leg.

4. Adjust your hand position on the strap so that your arms are extended and your hands are as close to your right foot as possible. Remember to keep your shoulders down.

5. Be aware of a tendency to arch your back. Keep your spine aligned against the mat (you may have to engage your abdominal muscles to do this). If you have discomfort in your lower back, try bending your left leg at the knee and placing the sole of your left foot on the mat. Bring your left heel toward your buttocks until you are comfortable in your lower back and your back is flat on the mat.

6. Work the stretch at the edge of your flexibility for several long, deep breaths. Since the hamstrings are such large muscles, they benefit from staying in this stretch a bit longer than the usual 30 seconds. Try to hold this pose for at least a full minute, preferably several minutes.

7. When you have completed the first phase of this posture, straighten your left leg so that it is flat on the mat, transfer both ends of the strap to your right hand, and slowly lower your right leg to the ground out to the right side of your body. Press your left

hip into the ground and keep both legs firm. Adjust the length of the strap if necessary in order to keep your right leg completely straight. You can rest your foot on a thick book or block if it does not touch the floor. Stretch your left arm perpendicular to the left side of your body.

8. Press your right heel away from your body, and keep the toes flexed toward your head. Breathe into this stretch and work at the edge of your flexibility. Keep your left leg engaged and extended along the mat and your left foot flexed. Hold for a full minute.

9. Lift your right leg back toward the ceiling, and then lower it to the mat. Take a few deep breaths, giving yourself a moment to experience how your right leg feels compared with your left leg.

10. Repeat on the left side.

KNEE TO CHEST POSE

The Knee to Chest pose massages the abdominal organs, relieves gas, and lengthens the muscles of the lower back and the upper legs. Combining Ujjayi breathing (see page 101) with the posture is especially helpful because the posture and breath act as a strong compressing force in the stimulation of the abdomen.

How to do the pose:

1. Lay on your back, legs extended and arms resting at your sides. Relax and surrender the weight of your body into the mat. Focus on your breath for three breaths.

2. On an exhalation, bring your left knee toward your chest. Wrap your hands on top of your folded knee. Keep your right leg straight and pressed against the mat with your foot flexed. Keep the

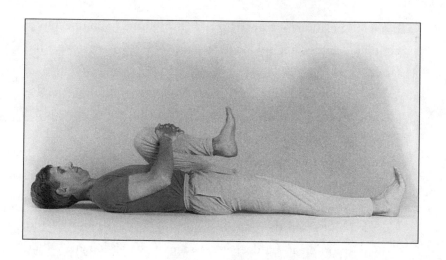

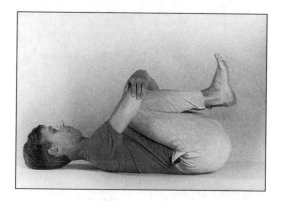

kneecap of your extended right leg lifted by tightening the thigh
muscle in the front.

3. Pull your left leg snugly to your chest, keeping your elbows tucked
   in toward your body, your shoulders relaxed on the mat.

4. Keep your back flat against the mat, your chin tucked, and the back
   of your neck elongated and pressed toward the mat.

5. Hold this position for several breaths. If you have room to explore, continue to press your folded left leg into your chest on your exhalations.

6. Extend your left leg back down to lay alongside your right leg. Notice the difference between the two legs and hip joints.

7. Repeat the posture on the right side.

8. Next bring both knees to your chest, pressing them against your body and massaging your abdominal organs. If you are flexible enough, you can lock the elbow joint of each arm over the front of each leg and grasp the opposite elbow with the opposite hand. This position creates a deeper massage of the abdomen. Otherwise, hold each knee with one hand.

9. Elongate the back by pressing out of the crown of your head and the base of your spine. Press your hips and spine into the mat, and the back of your neck toward the mat.

10. Finish by extending your legs and bringing your arms to your sides. Take a few breaths.

KNEE DOWN TWIST

The Knee Down Twist is a wonderful way to twist the spine, stretch the torso, and tone the waist. We don't often get a chance to move our spines in a twisting motion, so this pose aids in keeping us limber in every direction.

How to do the pose:

1. Lay flat on your back with your arms straight out to the sides so that your body forms a cross; palms face up, legs are straight and together.

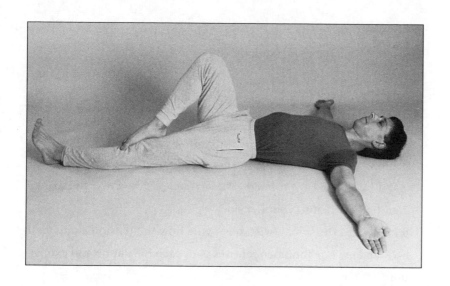

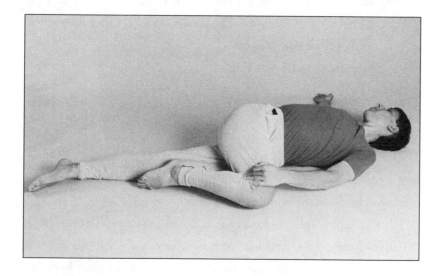

2. Inhaling, bend your right leg and place the sole of your right foot on
   top of your left knee.

3. Exhaling, turn your head to the right and lower your right knee across your left leg, pressing the knee toward the floor.

4. To enhance the spinal twist and stretch out your right hamstring and buttock muscle, you can place your left hand on your right knee and press the knee further toward the floor.

5. At the same time, press your right shoulder toward the mat. Depending on your flexibility, your right shoulder might come off the mat a bit as your right knee carries your weight across the axis of your body and onto your left side.

6. Breathe into the spinal twist, observing how the tension along your back and in your abdomen releases with each inhalation and exhalation.

7. After a few breaths, lift your right leg back to the center of your torso and straighten it out on the mat. Feel the full width of your back against the mat. Bring your awareness to your torso, feeling the difference between the two sides.

8. Repeat the twist on the left side.

CHILD POSE

The Child pose is a very relaxing way to spend a few minutes. This posture is particularly beneficial after a difficult pose or when you need a relaxation break in the middle of a stressful day.

The Child pose relieves lower back tension, increases circulation in the abdominal organs, and increases elasticity in the hip flexor muscles. If you feel too much pressure from the weight of your body on your knees, place a blanket underneath them and between your calf and thigh muscles for comfort and support. If you can't bend forward far enough to get your forehead to the mat, you can place a pillow or blanket between your chest and your thighs and one on the mat di-

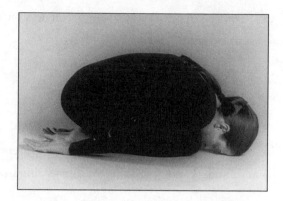

rectly under your forehead. This will ensure a very comfortable resting pose.

How to do the pose:

1. Sit on your mat with your legs folded under you and rest your buttocks on your heels. Close your eyes and take three long, deep breaths.
2. Exhaling, lower your torso forward so that your chest rests on your thighs and your forehead rests on the mat.
3. Relax your face, drop your shoulders, and soften your abdomen.
4. Feel the release at the top of your spine, between the shoulder blades, and allow your back to widen and relax.
5. Lay your arms alongside your body and let them rest heavily on the mat.
6. If you experience too much pressure in your head, bring your arms around in front of you, form fists, stack your fisted hands one on top of the other, and rest your forehead on them.
7. Hold the pose for several breaths, enjoying the relaxation.

8. To come out of the pose, simply roll up slowly, place your hands on your lap, and sit quietly.

FOREARM STRETCH

The Forearm Stretch opens and lengthens the insides of the forearms and also opens the shoulder joints. It helps relieve tension in the arms and shoulders and thus helps the arms swing freely while walking.

How to do the pose:

1. Start out on your hands and knees, with your hands aligned under your shoulders and your knees under your hips. Relax in this position for a minute, just breathing easily. Gradually sink back until your buttocks rest on your heels. Use a blanket or pillow under your knees if you feel too much stress in your knees from the weight of your body.
2. Instead of bending forward, as in the Child pose, place your palms flat on the mat with your fingers pointed back toward your knees and the insides of your forearms turned away from your chest.

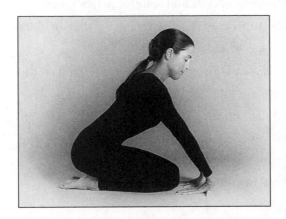

Stretch the insides of your forearms by pressing your palms down into the mat.

3. If you want to increase the stretch, keep your palms on the mat and lean your torso back toward your heels.
4. Take several long, deep breaths.
5. Release your hands and shake out your arms.

Sun Salutation *(Surya Namaskar)*

The Sun Salutation is a series of yoga postures coordinated with the breath that flow from pose to counterpose. It provides a challenging and energizing workout and is a great way to warm up all parts of the body before or after a walk. There are many variations of the Sun Salutation, and we have presented a basic variation here. In the beginning, stay in each pose for 10 to 30 seconds. Aim to extend gradually the number of breaths you take in each pose.

POSE 1: MOUNTAIN

The Mountain pose forms the basis for the Sun Salutation and is the starting and ending position. It is important to begin the series with proper alignment. Please read the following instructions carefully.

Feet

Your feet are the foundation for the Mountain pose, so it is important to place them properly. Stand with your feet together and planted firmly on your mat. Spread your toes by lifting them off the mat and lowering them back down, one at a time if possible. Lift the arches of your feet and distribute your weight evenly between the balls and heels of your feet, and the right and left sides of each foot. Bring your feet

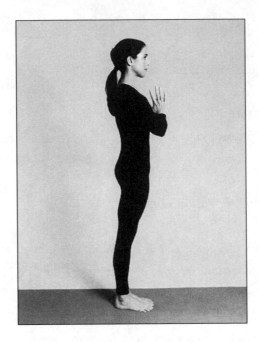

parallel to each other and, if possible, have your heels and big toes touching. If you are unable to bring your feet together so they are touching, stand with feet parallel, about 2 to 3 inches apart.

Legs

The strength and power of the Mountain pose is anchored in the legs, so it is important to keep your legs strong. Keep both ankles in line with each other, lift out of your heels, engage your calf and thigh muscles by pressing the muscles toward the bones. Lift your kneecaps and extend your legs upward.

Hips and Buttocks

Your tailbone is tucked under and your pubic bone pushed forward. Your pelvic girdle becomes level and square, so that the hipbones are facing forward like two headlights. Engage your buttocks muscles so they feel solid and strong. When you engage your leg and buttocks muscles in this way, you ensure that your lower back and torso muscles will be protected from injury.

Torso

Elongate by rising out of your waist and hips, lifting your sternum, opening your chest, and rolling your shoulders back and down. Place your hands in front of your heart in prayer position.

Head and Neck

Lengthen the back of your neck, bringing your chin parallel to the floor and pressing out of the crown of your head. Your head should feel like it is floating, loose and balanced atop your torso and legs.

Take three long, deep breaths and experience the strength of the Mountain pose, in which you are perfectly balanced, connected to earth and sky.

POSE 2: STANDING BACK BEND

Come into the Mountain pose at the front of your mat. Inhale and raise your arms above your head. Bring your palms together in prayer position with your elbows straight.

Arch your back slightly, keeping your feet firmly on the mat and grounding yourself through the strength of your legs and buttocks muscles. Think of your pelvis as your center of stability while your upper body reaches up and away from your solid stance. Remember to keep your leg and buttocks muscles engaged to support and protect your lower back. If you have a weak lower back, lower your arms and

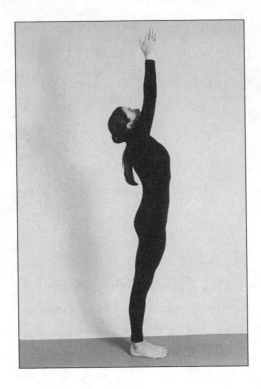

place your hands on your lower back for support as you arch slightly backward.

POSE 3: STANDING FORWARD BEND

From the Standing Back Bend, exhale and bend forward from the waist, rounding your back. Let the top of your head drop toward the mat. If possible, keep your legs straight without bending the knees. If you can, place your hands on the outsides of your feet with palms flat on the mat. Lift your kneecaps. Experience the intense stretch to the legs, buttocks, and back. Breathe deeply and hold for 10 seconds.

To ease the stretch in the backs of your legs, you can press your

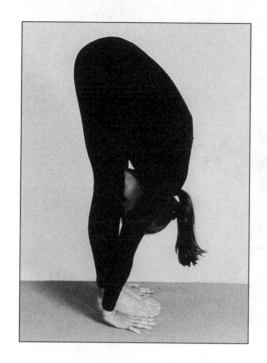

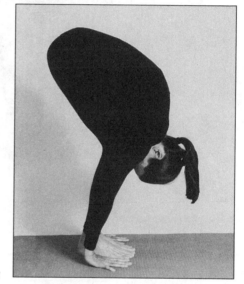

Alternate pose

heels into the mat slightly while lifting your toes. If you cannot touch the mat while keeping your legs straight, bend at the knees and rest your chest on your thighs; place your hands alongside the outsides of your feet, and touch the mat with your fingertips.

POSE 4: LEFT LUNGE

Next, inhale, lift your torso and extend your spine as you look up. Keep arms extended and fingertips touching the floor on either side of your

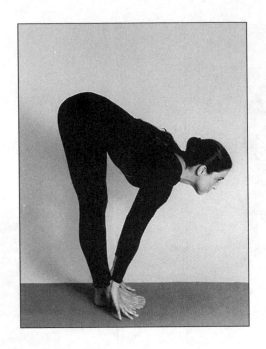

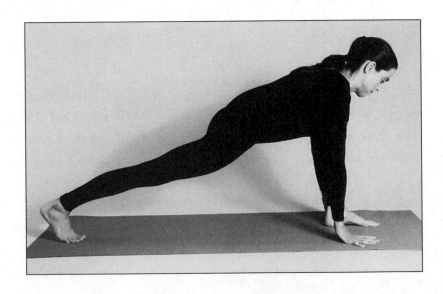

feet. Bend your knees if you cannot keep fingers in contact with the mat.

Exhaling, lower palms to the floor, extend your right leg behind you, toes touching the mat. Keep your left knee bent directly over your left foot. Your left thigh should be as parallel to the ground as possible. Your right leg will be straight behind you, with toes flexed. Push your chest slightly forward between your arms. Keep your face relaxed. If possible, there should be a straight line between your shoulders and your left heel. If this pose is too challenging for you to hold, you can rest your right knee on the ground.

POSE 5: PLANK

Inhaling, bring your left leg back alongside your right leg. Keep your arms straight and rigid, making sure your shoulders and upper arm bones are directly over your wrists. Also make sure your inner elbows are facing each other. Keep your back and buttocks in a straight line so

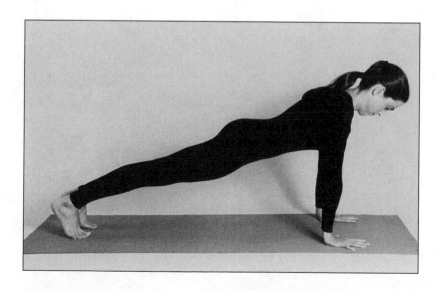

that your body forms an even, slanted line from head to feet. Keep the muscles in your shoulders and upper back strong, and engage your abdominal muscles by pressing the lower abs, just above the pubis, toward your spine.

POSE 6: EIGHT POINT

Exhaling, come out of the Plank pose by bending your knees to the mat, followed by your arms, your chest, and your chin. This transition may feel awkward at first, but with practice it will begin to flow smoothly. Your back will be arched, your buttocks raised. Keep your toes flexed and palms flat on floor directly under your shoulders. Look up. For a greater challenge, try the Alternate Four-Limbed Staff pose.

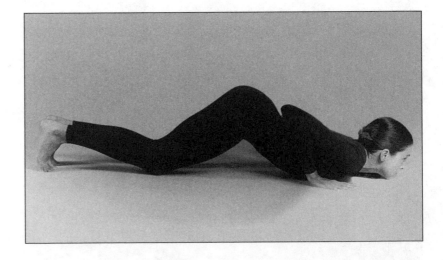

ALTERNATIVE POSE 6: ALTERNATE FOUR-LIMBED STAFF (YOGA PUSH-UP)

This position builds strength in the upper arms, shoulders, upper back, and chest. Be sure to engage your full-body muscular strength, being careful not to force yourself into the position by overstressing your shoulders, arms, and chest. As you move into the pose, keep the muscular engagement formed in the Plank pose.

Exhaling, lower yourself from the Plank pose by bending your arms and shifting slightly forward on your toes so that your elbows end up directly over your wrists. Keep your arms and elbows close to your body as you lower your chest and torso to several inches above the mat. Your hands and toes (which are still flexed) are the only body parts touching the mat, as if you were in a push-up.

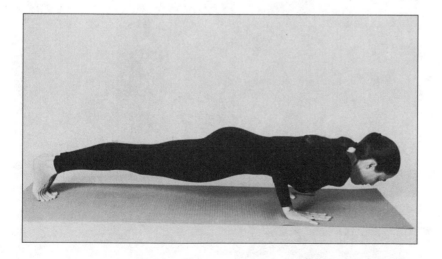

POSE 7: UPWARD DOG

Inhaling, press your weight into your hands, lower your hips, raise your chest, straighten your arms, arch your back, and lift your thighs and shins off the mat. Make sure your buttocks and thigh muscles are engaged and your chin is parallel to the mat. All your weight is distributed to your hands and feet; your legs are together, extending behind you. Shift your feet so that your weight is on the tops of the feet and your toes are no longer flexed. Broaden your chest and drop your shoulders away from your ears. Stretch your torso upward, extending your spine and the lift of your chest.

If you are unable to lift your legs off the mat completely, simply lower your knees to the mat.

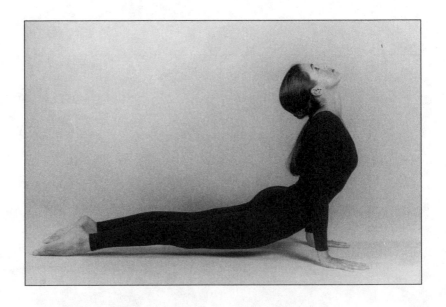

POSE 8: DOWNWARD DOG

Exhaling, flex your feet, keep your legs straight and lift your hips up and back. Once you are in position, your body will look like an upside-down V shape. Keeping your feet parallel to each other, lower your heels toward the mat. If this position stretches your calves and ham-strings too intensely in the beginning, keep your heels off the mat. Press your weight evenly into your hands and feet, stretch your arms fully, and press your sternum toward the mat and your torso toward your legs.

Tighten the muscles of your thighs by hugging them to the thigh-bones and draw your kneecaps in and up. Keep your back straight. As you tilt your tailbone up, press back into your hips and lift your but-tocks toward the ceiling. This movement facilitates maximum length-ening of your arms, torso, and legs. Let your head hang, and make sure your neck and shoulders are relaxed.

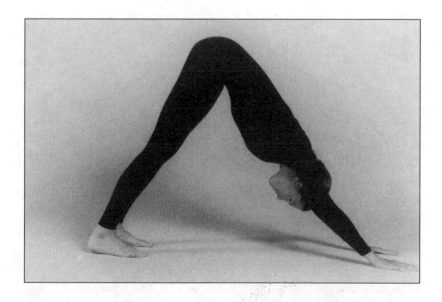

Note: The Downward Dog can be done on its own and is very beneficial for the body. It slows the heartbeat, helps open the shoulders,
tones and stretches the legs, and strengthens the wrists and ankles. It is
a very soothing posture for the mind as well. You can also rest your
forehead on a pillow for deeper relaxation.

POSE 9: RIGHT LUNGE

Inhaling, shift your weight onto your palms, bend your knees, and
swing your right knee forward. Place your right foot on the mat centered between your shoulders, keeping your right knee in line with
your right ankle, your right shin perpendicular to the mat. Keep your
right thigh as parallel to the mat as possible. Your left leg will be
straight behind you, your left foot flexed and resting on the toes and
ball. If you cannot keep your palms flat, rest on your fingertips.

Push your chest slightly forward between your arms. Keep your face

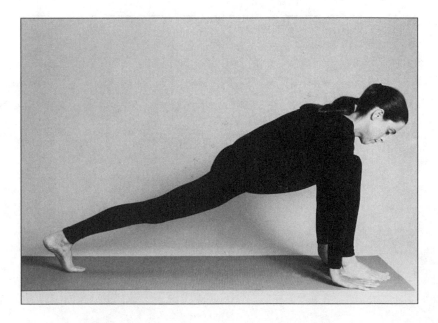

soft and relaxed. There should be a straight line between your shoulders and your right foot.

POSE 10: STANDING FORWARD BEND

Exhaling, bring your left leg forward, placing your feet together, and raise your hips toward the ceiling. This is the same Standing Forward Bend described in Pose 3. Bend forward from the waist with your back rounded, tucking your tailbone under as you fold your torso down toward your thighs. If possible, keep your legs straight, without bending the knees.

Place your hands along the outsides of your feet with palms flat on your mat. To ease the stretch in the backs of your legs, you can press your heels into the mat while slightly lifting your toes. If you cannot touch the mat while keeping your legs straight, bend your knees, rest-

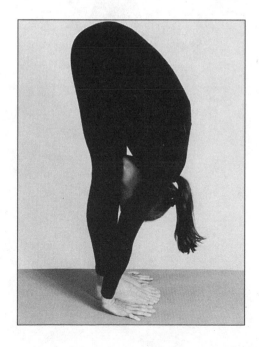

ing your chest on your thighs, and place your hands on the mat along the outsides of your feet. You can also touch the floor with your finger-tips or rest your hands on your shins. Stretch and open your thighs, lift your kneecaps. Notice the increased flexibility and energy in your legs and back.

POSE 11: STANDING BACK BEND

We're about to complete the cycle now. Inhaling, lift your hands off the mat. Keep your back rounded as you lift your torso. Tighten your buttocks muscles to protect your lower back as you come up. Stretch your arms all the way over your head, bending back from the hips. Bring your palms together. Look up at your hands. Stay centered, keep-

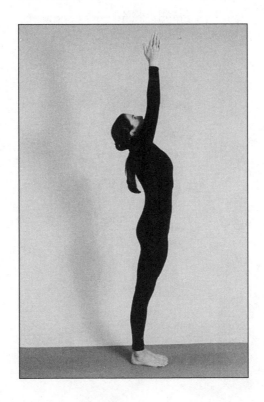

ing your hips directly over your feet, your thigh muscles engaged, and your pubic bone pushed forward.

POSE 12: MOUNTAIN

Exhaling, let your arms come back into prayer position, palms together in front of your heart. Pause here. Close your eyes, relax your face, and notice the sensations all over your body. Appreciate the feeling of energy and peace that's within you. Take several deep breaths and start the series again, this time lunging with the left leg first.

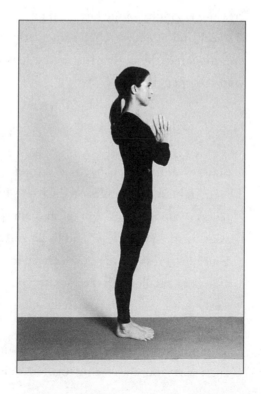

Standing Postures

Beginners: We start all the standing postures in the Mountain pose with instructions to stand with your feet together. If you are unable to bring your feet together so they are touching, stand with your feet parallel, about 2 to 3 inches apart.

WARRIOR

The powerful Warrior pose fills the body with a sense of nobility and strength. It helps develop strength and endurance, while the limbs and torso receive a vigorous workout. The Warrior pose is excellent for increasing flexibility in the knee and hip joints and relieving stiffness in the neck and shoulders. It is a particularly good posture for walkers because it strengthens all parts of the legs and buttocks muscles and works to open the hips.

How to do the pose:

1. Stand with your feet together. Center your hips directly over your feet. Tighten the muscles on the fronts of your thighs and tuck your tailbone under (this will push your pubic bone forward). Lift your torso equally, front and back, and lengthen your spine out of your hips. Press the top of your head toward the ceiling and let your chin float parallel with the mat. Rest your arms at your sides. Breathe easily until you feel both feet squarely on the mat and a solid, grounded sense in your center.
2. Take a big step to the right so that your legs are spread 3 to 4 feet apart with your toes facing forward. Bend your arms, bringing your

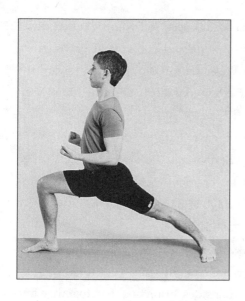

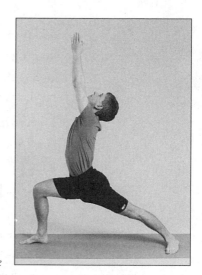

Alternate pose

elbows close to your waist, and form fists with your hands. Keep your forearms parallel to the mat.

3. Turn your right foot out 90 degrees, and keep your left foot perpendicular to your right foot. Turn your torso to the right in line with your right knee.

4. Exhaling, bend your right knee. Stretch both sides of your torso up equally, and roll your tailbone under. If possible, lower your pelvis until your right shin is perpendicular to the mat. Your right knee and ankle should be in line with each other. It is very important to keep them well aligned to prevent injury; extending the knee past the ankle puts too much stress on the knee. Bring your right thigh as close to parallel to the mat as you can. Keep your left leg energized and strong by pushing down on the outside of your left foot, keeping it in contact with the mat. Engage your buttocks muscles and hips. For beginners, hold this position for a count of 10.

5. For a more challenging stretch, inhale as you sweep your arms up overhead, bringing your hands into prayer position. Take care not to

raise your shoulders. Broaden your chest, roll your shoulders down and back, and extend your spine up and out of your pelvis. Keep your chin and face relaxed. Press the top of your head toward the ceiling. Stretch fully upward from your left heel to the top of your fingertips.

6. Breathe fully, opening your rib cage. Extending your spine toward your fingers, keeping your chest broad and your shoulders rolled back and down, continue to lower your hips slightly with every exhalation, bringing your right thigh as parallel to the mat as you can. Hold the pose for 10 to 30 seconds.

7. To come up, inhale and press your weight into your right foot, lifting your hips until both legs are straight. Turn your torso and feet forward; lower your arms to your sides; bring your feet together; and close your eyes, taking a moment to experience the warrior strength building in your body.

8. Repeat on the left side.

Beginners: If your thighs are not strong enough at first, you can practice this posture with your hands on your bent thigh, making it easier to balance and support yourself.

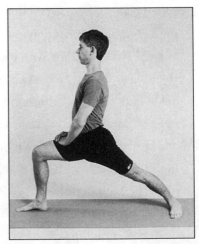

Alternate pose

TREE POSE

The Tree pose is a wonderful teacher of stability and balance. It develops the power of concentration, strengthens the equilibrium, and promotes character and willpower. Practicing this pose will also give you a better sense of balance when you walk and will strengthen the quadriceps muscles of the thighs to help prevent knee pain.

How to do the pose:

1. Stand in the Mountain pose with both feet together and your hips centered directly over your feet. Tighten the muscles on the fronts of your thighs and tuck your tailbone under, which will push your pubic bone forward. Tighten your buttocks muscles and lengthen your spine out of your hips. Lift your torso equally front and back, press the top of your head toward the ceiling, and let your chin float parallel with the mat. Breathe easily until you feel both feet squarely on the ground and a solid, grounded sense in your center.

2. Inhaling, shift your weight to your left leg and lift your right foot a few inches off the mat. For better balance, spread the toes of your left foot, evenly distribute your weight on that foot, and keep your left inner heel grounded.

3. Exhaling, bend your right leg, clasping the ankle with your right hand and placing the sole flush against the inside of your left thigh. Although you will eventually want to place your foot as high as you can, when you start out it can be placed just above the knee, on the calf, or on the ankle. Opening your hips, extend your right knee out to the side.

4. To develop balance, focus on a point on the floor or wall in front of you, keeping your gaze fixed on that spot.

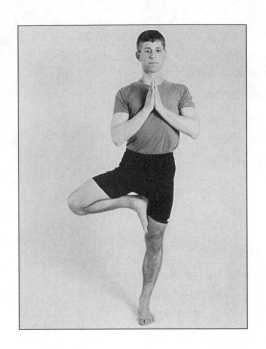

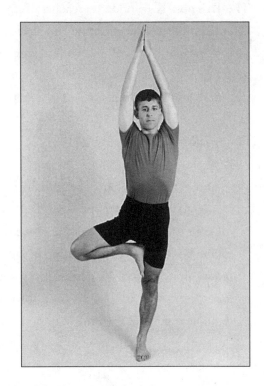

5. Place your hands in front of your heart in the prayer position. As you gain steadiness in the posture, you can raise your arms above your head with your palms pressed against each other. In the beginning, you can also place your hands on your hips for more stability.

6. Maintain a sense of strength and stability in your left leg, keeping the foot firmly planted on the mat, the knee straight, and the thigh firm. Try to gain lift and extension from your foot through the whole length of your spine to the top of your head.

7. At the same time, survey your posture to make sure your hips are square and open, buttocks firm, tailbone tucked in, and the front of

your torso lifted and strong. Drop your right knee away from the hip and push it toward the back, opening the hips further. Roll your shoulders down and back, opening up your chest.

8. Because this pose is challenging, it is easy for the shoulders to hunch up. Keep them relaxed. Soften your face, nose, and throat as well.

9. Hold your balance for 10 to 30 seconds. When you are ready, let your arms float gently down to your sides and return to the Mountain pose. Experience the calm, steady balance that results from the Tree pose.

10. Repeat on the other side.

Floor Postures

LOCUST POSE

The Locust pose builds strength in the lower back and improves flexibility along the entire spine. Since walking can tend to compress the lower back, the Locust is wonderful support for a walking practice.

How to do the pose:

1. Lie on your stomach with your forehead on the mat and your hands alongside your torso, palms down.

2. Inhale and engage your buttocks and lower back muscles while lifting your legs and upper torso off the mat. Lift your hands and arms off the mat, and use this motion to enhance the lift of your upper torso. Look up toward the ceiling.

3. While in the pose, constantly try to lift your upper legs and chest

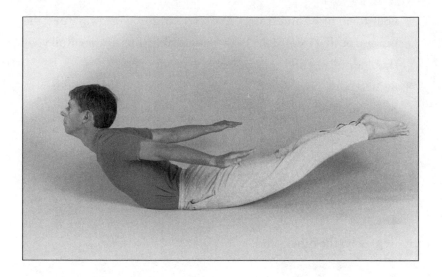

further from the mat. Stretch the fronts of your thighs and point your toes behind you.

4. Breathe deeply in the posture. You may notice that your body rocks a little with the incoming and outgoing breath. Hold the posture for 10 to 30 seconds.

5. Come out of the posture with an exhalation and lie flat again, with your head resting on one side or the other. Repeat the pose.

Beginners: If you are unable to lift your chest and legs off the ground simultaneously, practice lifting your chest while keeping your legs on the mat and then lifting your legs while your chest remains on the mat.

COBRA POSE

Practicing the Cobra pose will increase strength, flexibility, and alignment in the spine and improve posture. The arms, wrists, and back muscles are strengthened; the chest opens and the rib cage expands, helping to increase the capacity of the lungs. This pose is a great way to prepare the body for walking in a free and easy manner.

How to do the pose:

1. Begin by lying on your belly, resting your forehead on the mat. Let your chest, stomach, thighs, and knees feel weighty against the mat. Relax the small of your back. Keep your legs together, feet touching. The tops of your feet should be flat against the mat—they should not be flexed. Lengthen your body by pressing the crown of your head away from your feet.

2. Bend your elbows, and place your hands flat on the mat, directly beneath your shoulders, with the fingers spread wide. Make sure your elbows remain at your sides throughout the pose. Broaden your chest and roll your shoulder blades down and back. Press your hipbones and pubic bone into the mat.

3. Inhaling, engage your lower back and buttocks muscles and use their

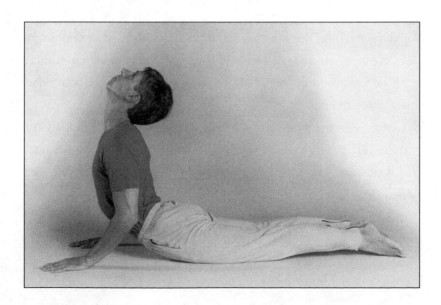

strength to lift your head, shoulders, and chest off the floor. Use the strength of your back and spine to generate and maintain the lift rather than relying on your arms. When you do take some of your weight onto your hands, keep your arms bent, your elbows close to the body, and your shoulders dropped away from your ears.

4. Lift your chest and belly until just your pubic bone is in contact with the mat. Continue to tighten your buttocks and thigh muscles, push your pubic bone toward the mat, and press your weight into your hands and legs. Your feet will tend to come apart; pressing them together will help you to keep the buttocks muscles engaged.

5. Extend your spine from its base to the top of your skull, and use the spinal muscles to keep the stretch alive. Lengthen the back of your neck and press out of the crown of your head. Look up slightly. Don't let the posture become static while you are extending.

6. While in the posture, gently press down into your hands while pulling them toward your hips. The hands don't actually move, but this pull assists in the upward extension of your spine and the stretching of your chest and abdomen. You can actually feel the skin on your stomach stretching.

7. Exhale and hold this position for 10 to 30 seconds. Scan your body for tension, letting your face and throat relax. Bring your attention to the expansion in your chest and heart area and to the continued extension of your spine.

8. Come out of the pose slowly, bending your arms and releasing your spine vertebra by vertebra, feeling the spine adjust back to its normal curvature. Rest for a moment on the mat or in Child pose (see page 56).

YOGA MUDRA

This is one of the most relaxing of all the yoga postures and when practiced gives a sense of meditation in motion. The ease of the movement
allows you to focus primarily on the breath, helping you sink deeply
into relaxation. Yoga Mudra tones the abdominal muscles, gives a deep
stretch to the shoulders, triceps, and biceps muscles, and soothes the
central nervous system.

How to do the pose:

1. Sit on your heels with your legs bent under you. Place a blanket between your thighs and calf muscles for comfort if sitting on your
   heels is too uncomfortable or if you have weak or injured knees. Rest

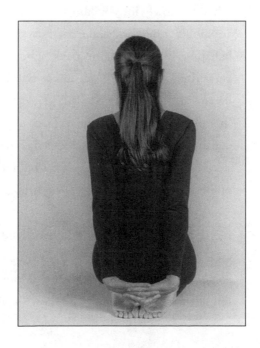

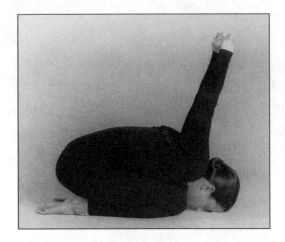

your palms on your knees. Extend your spine up from the hips, keeping your chin parallel to the mat, lengthening the back of your neck, and pressing out of the top of your head.

2. Inhaling, slowly lift your arms straight out in front of you until they are shoulder height, parallel to the mat.

3. Exhaling, bring your arms back behind you and interlace your fingers. Keep your arms straight and roll your shoulders back and down. Take a moment to adjust to the stretch in your arms and shoulders. If you are unable to bring your hands together, wrap one end of a tie or strap around each hand. This will allow you to straighten and then lift your arms behind you, increasing the range of motion in your shoulders. The strap should be taut between your hands.

4. On an exhalation, lower your torso and head toward the mat and raise your arms behind you toward the ceiling. Rest your forehead gently on the mat. If you can't bend forward far enough to get your forehead to the mat, place a pillow or blanket between your chest

and your thighs and one on the mat directly under your forehead. Once in the full position, use your breath to help you relax into the stretch. Stay in the pose for 10 to 30 seconds, gradually increasing your holding time as you are comfortable.

5. Inhaling, very slowly lift your head and torso back into a sitting position, keeping your arms straight and engaged behind you.

6. Exhaling, release your hands and allow them to float back to a resting position on your thighs.

FORWARD BEND

The Forward Bend has a powerful healing effect. It stretches the body from the top of the head to the soles of the feet and gives an intense stretch to the whole length of the spine, helping to increase the flow of the life force throughout the body. The Forward Bend rests and massages the heart, improves digestion, tones the kidneys, bladder, and pancreas, stimulates the entire reproductive system, and relieves sciatica.

When you practice, move slowly and hold the posture for at least 1 to 2 minutes so you can experience the deep stretch to the whole back side of the body.

How to do the pose:

1. Begin by sitting with your legs extended on the mat, heels pushed away and toes flexed, back toward your body. Feel your buttocks firm against the floor. If you shift your weight from side to side, you will feel your sit bones. Make sure your weight is evenly distributed between them.

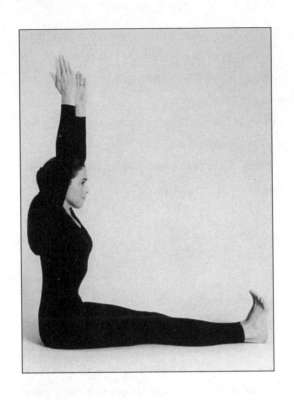

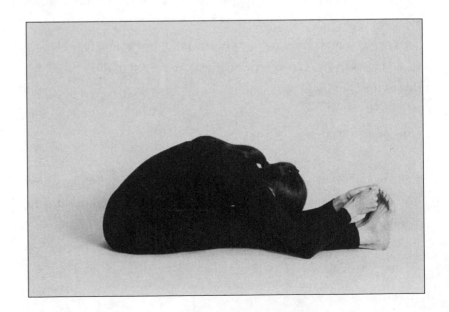

walking yoga

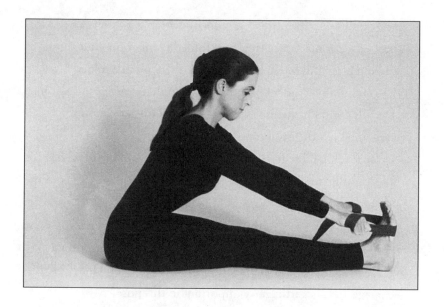

2. Inhaling, raise your arms toward the ceiling, extend your spine out of your hips and your head upward from your shoulders without raising the shoulders.

3. Keep the backs of your legs pressed down and the backs of your knees open and pressed into the mat. Keep your thighs and backs of your knees pressed firmly into the mat during the entire pose. You may need to use a strap to support your efforts to keep the backs of your legs flat on the mat. Take the strap and wrap it around the balls of your feet. Wrap the ends of the strap around your hands so that your arms are extended straight out from your shoulders and your hands are as close to your feet as possible. Keeping your legs flat on the mat in this pose is more important than reaching your forehead to your legs.

4. Exhaling, bend forward, keeping your back slightly rounded while moving your torso forward and down toward the thighs. Stretch forward from your waist and, eventually, rest your forehead on your

knees. Relax into the pose. If it is uncomfortable for you to bend forward, you can place a bolster or a folded blanket on your thighs to rest your arms and forehead on. You can also place a folded blanket, a few inches thick, under your buttocks so that you are sitting on its edge. This will lift the hips slightly, making the stretch in the backs of your legs a little less intense.

5. As you develop more flexibility, you can grasp your big toes with the thumb and first two fingers of each hand. Keep your elbows to the sides and off the mat.

6. Make every effort to lengthen your spine and stretch it from its base to the top of your head. Continue to let your lower back open and release. Keep your abdomen soft. Taking long, deep Ujjayi breaths (see page 101) is particularly important in this pose.

7. Come out of the pose by lifting your upper body off your legs and stretching upward with your arms. Create a concave arch in your back as you lift, then pause for a moment with your arms stretched upward, back arched, and sternum open. Then exhale and allow your arms to drop to the sides of your body.

CORPSE POSE (YOGA NIDRA)

We always suggest ending your yoga sequence with a relaxation experience called the Corpse pose or *Yoga Nidra*. *Yoga Nidra* means "yogic sleep," and of all the gifts yoga offers, the emphasis on relaxation may be its most beneficial. Practicing the deep relaxation technique of the Corpse pose is often more of a challenge for people than engaging in the more active postures. We have been so habituated to doing instead of just being that the thought of lying still may seem foreign and strange. For some of us, it can be uncomfortable to let go and remain quiet because when we relax and stay still, unfinished thoughts and feelings may surface. When you practice the yogic technique of deep

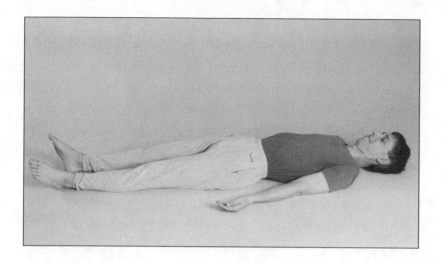

relaxation, the body is allowed to sink into a peaceful, calm state in which the mind becomes serene and quiet.

Try not to skip the Corpse pose, even if you feel you have limited time for your walking yoga session. This pose is vital for bringing the essence of yoga into your everyday life, and it has a powerful rejuvenating effect on the body, mind, and spirit. More than being a tool for relieving stress, the Corpse pose provides appropriate closure for your yoga practice. Taking the time to experience stillness; letting the blood flow normally again; and respecting the fact that it takes a while for energy to shift, for the sensations in the body and the thoughts of the mind to sort themselves out, is of deep importance to your walking yoga practice.

How to do the pose:

1. Lie on your back with your eyes closed and your arms on the mat beside your body, palms facing down.

2. Bend your legs at the knees and place your feet flat on the mat. Lift your hips toward the ceiling and arch your back. Stretch out the back of your neck, tuck your chin under, and begin to lower your back toward the floor vertebra by vertebra. The idea is to extend the spine fully so that you can keep it flat on the mat. Take your time. If you have discomfort in your lower back, you may find that placing a pillow or a bolster under the backs of your knees helps your back to relax more.

3. Once you are lying flat on the mat again, stretch your body from head to toe by pressing your feet away from your head. Relax your legs, allowing them to roll gently apart and to the sides. Your knees and toes will fall out to the sides as well.

4. Relax your arms alongside your body about one to two feet from your torso, palms facing up. Release the tension in your neck by rolling your head from side to side and pressing your shoulders down, away from your ears.

5. Breathing deeply, slowly scan your body, starting at your feet and moving to the top of your head. Pause when you sense fatigue, tension, or stress, and direct the breath to these areas. Each time you exhale, consciously relax that part of your body, visualizing the tension and fatigue draining away. Visualize a healing light moving through your body in waves, each wave attuned to the motion of the breath. Everywhere the light touches, visualize letting go into a deeper place of integration.

6. Once you have taken this journey, imagine that your body is becoming very heavy. Feel the sensation of your mat and the floor underneath supporting each part of your body. Sink into your mat, and deeply and completely relax. Allow any residual tension to be released as your breath comes in and goes out, gradually becoming more shallow.

7. Watch your inhalations and exhalations, focusing only on the

sound of your breath. As your mind wanders, gently bring your awareness back to the breath, focusing on the sound it makes, its rhythm, the way it fills your lungs and belly. Whenever your thoughts arise, watch them appear in your mind, acknowledge them, and send them drifting away with your exhalation. Yogic sleep is conscious rest, so keep your mind awake yet relaxed.

8. Practice this pose for at least 5 minutes. Use a timer if worrying about the time will distract you from relaxing. If you have time and your walking yoga practice has been particularly vigorous, practice this pose for 10 to 15 minutes.

9. Come out of the Corpse pose slowly. Wiggle your fingers and toes. Move your awareness to the room, recalling where you are. Concentrate on keeping the mind quiet.

10. Bend your knees; roll over on your side and rest for a moment. Then bring yourself slowly to a seated position. There is no hurry. Sit here, savoring the experience before you come to standing and move into the rest of your day. We recommend softly chanting *aum* before you get up from your yoga mat, because the sound will harmonize all parts of you and remind you of the eternal nature of your spirit.

Chapter 4

the practice of
walking yoga

Recently we were in New York City, on Fifth Avenue just south of Central Park. We had finished meeting with a speaking coach to help us prepare our talk for a large group of yoga practitioners at a conference, and now we were hungry and looking for a place to eat. It was around two in the afternoon, and the streets were filled with people. Everyone was hurrying to a destination and seemed preoccupied with inner thoughts. You know the scene—it's where the expression "rat race" comes from. Many of the faces we saw looked tense, irritated, or defeated, whole bodies armored against connection or contact with anyone or anything. You've experienced this type of walking. Even though your body is moving, you are miles away, thinking, planning, worrying, wrestling with some problem or another, just present enough to get where you are going in one piece.

Walking can be so much more, no matter where you are or what you need to do. Walking is a doorway to being in your body instead of your head, experiencing instead of thinking. When you walk with awareness, you can regroup and return to your center, clear your thoughts and feelings, and align your inner and outer worlds. It's a time when you can be a natural animal as well as a socialized member of society—when you can be on the earth feeling both your primal and your eternal nature. Most important, walking can be a time to regain your perspective and to experience yourself as healthy, integrated, and alive.

How do you develop the capacity for this experience? The key is to approach walking as a full experience, not just a means of getting from one place to another. In yoga it is said that true yoga is "being there." In other words, when we are fully present, no matter what we are doing, we are doing a form of yoga.

Yogis say that none of us can really be present unless we are fully in our bodies. Your body is the one thing that is always firmly located in time and space—here and now. "Being here now" starts with coming home to your body. Awareness of your body is like an anchor that keeps the ship from drifting away from its place of safe harbor.

As humans, we are naturally conditioned to notice things that move and change. This is one of the reasons television is so popular and entertaining. There's always some new program or set of images coming on. We wouldn't have much interest in television if it showed the same image all the time. This natural conditioning probably developed as an aid to survival. Our ancestors living on the African savanna were more likely to survive when they were closely observant of the changes around them. So when we walk, it's easiest to stay present if we pay attention to things that are always changing. And the place to start is the breath.

Walking and the Breath

The breath is always moving and changing, expanding on the inhalations and contracting on the exhalations. Breathing is the power behind all our movement and is the source of our stamina and vitality. A good way to understand the connection between breath and vitality is to see how often we need to breathe. Every other bodily function in life—eating, drinking, digestion, and elimination—can be delayed, but not the breath. Go without a drink for two hours and you may not even notice it, but stop breathing, even for a few seconds, and you start to focus on it pretty quickly.

In addition, no other automatic system in the body, such as the heartbeat and the digestive processes, is as affected by your state of mind. When you get angry, your breath becomes both shallow and rapid, and when you are relaxed, your breath becomes slow and deep. Did your mother ever tell you to take ten deep breaths before you acted when you became angry, or has a friend advised you to "calm down and just take a few deep breaths"? This is good advice. Consciously taking long, deep breaths when you are angry dissipates the tense anxiety of the state, allowing you to think more clearly. The breath affects the mind and the mind affects the breath.

Yogis recognized that we are both spiritual and physical beings, and they considered the breath the link between the subtle experience of energy and spirit, and the denser experience of the physical body. The way we use language points to how the breath is a bridge between the inner life and the outer life, in both Western and Eastern cultures. In the West, when we feel most alive and filled with vitality, we call ourselves *inspired*, which translated from the Greek means "filled with spirit." When all energy leaves us and we pass from this life, we *expire* or die. Taking in a full breath is also called *inspiration*, and letting a breath out is called *expiration*. In yoga, breathing exercises are called *pranayamas*, which means "control of the vital energy." So when you consciously pay attention to your breath and control the flow of air, you are also controlling something more subtle and profound: your own life force.

Whenever you walk, pay attention to your breath. You can feel it coming in and going out with every few steps. Let this awareness be the start of your experience, first the breath, then the step. The conscious use of the breath is what distinguishes walking yoga from other forms of exercise. Your breath is the primary experience and the power behind your movement, both gross movements of the body and subtle movements of the mind and emotions. One way to understand this practice is to remember how filmmakers use the sound of the breath to dominate a scene when they want to create an especially thrilling or scary feeling. You are watching the images move, but the sound of the breath is the overriding experience. When you practice absorbing yourself in the breath as you walk, it feels the same way, you are walking and thinking, but the breath is the overriding sensation.

Conscious Breathing

Most of us learn to breathe only through the upper part of our lungs, causing a kind of shallow, rapid form of breathing. In addition, from a young age we are taught to hold in our stomachs, which inhibits deep breathing and reinforces our inclination toward chest breathing. Consequently, the lower lobes of the lungs, where most of the blood and oxygen exchange happens, are not sufficiently ventilated and the body doesn't receive enough oxygen and energy, or effectively eliminate toxins trapped in the lungs. Unfortunately, our shallow chest breathing feels most natural to us, so we have to relearn how to breathe fully.

Have you ever watched a child breathe when she is sleeping? Her lungs move in three parts each time she takes a breath. First, her tummy rises, then her ribs expand, and finally her shoulders lift as the tops of the lungs fill. A full breath for an adult should be exactly the same.

You may notice that your first attempts at these breathing exercises are a bit jerky and unsteady. You may also feel that you can't get enough air when you practice breathing consciously. Not to worry, with regular practice you can learn to use the full capacity of your lungs so that your breath becomes natural and deep. We recommend beginning your conscious breathing practice with the first and most important part of the complete yogic breath, abdominal breathing.

ABDOMINAL BREATHING

1. Start your practice sitting in a chair with a firm seat. Sit slightly forward so that your back is not resting against the back of the chair.
2. Place your feet flat on the floor, parallel to each other, your knees directly over your ankles, your lower legs perpendicular to the floor.
3. Tuck your tailbone under or toward the pubic bone, engage your buttocks and abdominal muscles, and straighten your back by lengthening out of the waist.
4. Roll your shoulders back and down, and lengthen the back of your neck. Bring your chin parallel to the floor and press upward out of the crown of your head.

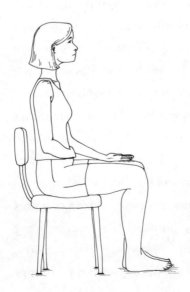

5. Relax your face. Place your left hand palm up on your left thigh and your right palm on your belly immediately below the belly button.
6. Exhale completely.
7. As you inhale through the nose, focus on your abdomen and notice how your hand moves away from your body as the lower lungs fill and moves back toward your body as you exhale. You can even exaggerate the expansion of the belly by pushing it out as you breathe in and then pressing it in as you breathe out.

Practice this breath for at least 10 inhalations and exhalations, preferably with your eyes closed to help you focus on the sensations and mechanics of the breath.

COMPLETE YOGIC BREATHING

The breath is central to the effectiveness of a walking yoga practice, and the key is to learn to breathe with the whole of your lungs. In yoga, this is referred to as complete yogic breathing. Before you begin, it will be helpful to understand what happens when you take a complete breath.

Think of the chest cavity as a cylinder. You can increase the volume of the cylinder in three ways: extend the floor of the cylinder down, expand the walls out, and move the top of the cylinder up. When you inhale in a complete breath, as oxygen flows into the bottoms of the lungs, your diaphragm muscle pushes down on the abdominal organs and your tummy expands. When you fill the middle parts of your lungs with air, your rib cage expands, increasing the volume of the cylinder of your chest. When you finish the breath by filling the top parts of your lungs, your collarbones, or clavicles, rise slightly to lengthen the cylinder of the chest and accommodate even more air. You know you are breathing the complete yogic breath when you can feel all three of

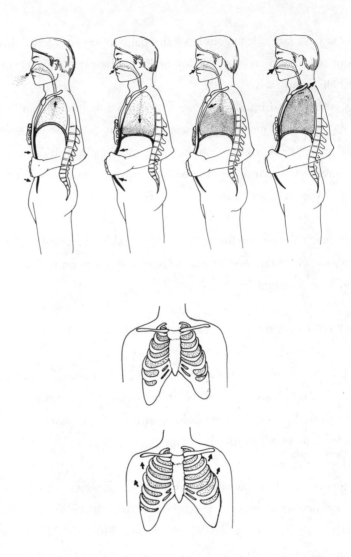

the movements: belly expanding, ribs moving out, and clavicles rising. When exhaling, you reverse the process and finish by using your abdominal muscles to press in on the internal organs in order to push up the diaphragm and expel the breath fully. A deep inhalation starts with a full exhalation.

■ ■ ■

How to practice the complete yogic breath:

1. Lie on your back on a blanket and relax your body completely.
2. Place one hand, palm down, on the center of your chest and the other on the center of your belly.
3. If at all possible, breathe through your nose on both the inhalation and the exhalation.
4. Exhale completely.
5. As you inhale, you will notice the hand on your belly rising as the diaphragm flattens and the lower lungs fill.
6. As the lungs continue to fill, the rib cage expands and the chest rises, moving the hand on your chest upward.
7. When your lungs take in their maximum capacity of oxygen, the clavicles or collarbones lift.
8. For a short moment, hold your breath in, and as you begin to exhale consciously, notice the collarbones lower, the chest fall, the rib cage contract, and finally the belly lower as the diaphragm moves back into its relaxed position.
9. Repeat for five breaths.

A tip for practice: You can use the image of pouring liquid into a container and watching the container fill from the bottom to the top. Visualize your torso as a container and instead of pouring liquid, pour air. As you inhale, the oxygen pours into the lungs, filling them from the bottom up, and as you exhale, the lungs empty from the top down.

You can practice the complete yogic breath when you first wake up in the morning, before you go to sleep at night, or during and after your daily yoga stretching routine.

Using the complete yogic breath when you walk not only helps to draw you into the sensation of breathing but also increases the overall vitality and energy available to you. You are taking in more oxygen with each breath, so each of your cells is getting more oxygen. And if you use your abdominal muscles to push in your tummy, you will also be getting rid of more of the stale carbon dioxide often trapped deep in the lungs. Tests performed on long-distance runners show that their maximum oxygen consumption rate, which measures the amount of oxygen a person can take in and transport to the various tissues of the body, increased by up to 50 percent through aerobic exercise. The increase depends on many factors, such as ventilation of the lungs, pumping capacity of the heart, and transfer of oxygen to the tissues. When you practice the complete yogic breath and all aspects of walking yoga, particularly the full-on-walking practice found on page 122, you will be able to increase your oxygen consumption rate. Your body's aerobic system will be able to work more efficiently, and your general fitness level will improve.

The complete yogic breath acts like a bellows in a blacksmith's forge. When the bellows moves up and down in great sweeps, the air blows across the coals and the coals burn hotter and brighter to produce the energy for the blacksmith to perform his job. You can feel this same process happen inside you as you oxygenate your body with the complete yogic breath. The body's fuel comes from the carbohydrates, fats, and proteins we eat, which are broken down and stored in the cells as nutrient fuel. It takes oxygen to burn the nutrient fuel and release energy into the system. When you consciously practice the complete yogic breath while walking, you infuse your lungs with fresh, oxygenated air, enhancing their effectiveness for "burning" fuel and providing you with energy and vitality.

UJJAYI BREATHING

Yogis practice a technique called Ujjayi breathing, which creates a rhythmic, soothing, oceanlike sound with each breath. This breathing exercise enhances the ventilation of the lungs, removes mucus, calms the nerves, and promotes relaxation and meditation. It is also helpful in reducing cravings and is an excellent tool to help you quit smoking. Fortunately, it is easy to learn.

How to practice Ujjayi breathing:

1. Imagine you have a mirror in front of you and you want to fog it up with your breath.
2. Open your mouth and exhale onto the imaginary mirror.
3. Practice this step until you can feel yourself making a small constriction in the back of your throat. Now close your mouth and create the same effect while breathing through your nose.
4. Focus on the back of your throat, and constrict the air passage a little bit as you inhale and exhale.
5. Practice the Ujjayi breath, taking the air in and out through your nose for 5 minutes.

When you control the flow of the breath in this way, the breath has a rasping quality and makes the sound you hear when you put a conch shell next to your ear. If you are having trouble with Ujjayi breathing, try this: Imagine you are a dog who is letting an intruder know he is alert by making a deep growling sound in the throat with your mouth closed. Ujjayi breathing is done just like that, only you don't constrict your throat so much that the sound actually becomes a growl.

We recommend using Ujjayi breathing as often as possible. During hatha yoga, Ujjayi breathing helps you quiet your mind and focus on the movement of the postures because of its soothing sound. This simple breath also helps facilitate relaxation in the postures. We use the Ujjayi breath during our walks, particularly during contemplative walking. You can actually train yourself to relax as soon as you hear the sound of your breath.

KAPALABHATI BREATHING

Kapalabhati is a Sanskrit word. *Kapal* means "skull," and *bhati* means "light" or "luster." Practice of this breathing exercise helps stimulate the brain and energize the body. It also helps clear the sinuses and lungs and strengthens the diaphragm, heart, and nervous system. The abdominal muscles are toned, and the energy or "fire in the belly" is activated.

Also known as breath of fire, Kapalabhati breathing is a simple exercise consisting of a quick and powerful exhalation followed by a passive inhalation. The exercise is done by using the diaphragm and the abdominal muscles to exhale forcefully through the nasal passages as if you were trying to clear something from your nose. The inhalation is automatic.

How to practice Kapalabhati breathing:

1. Sit in a comfortable position, either in a chair or on a mat.
2. Use a tissue to clear your nasal passages before starting.
3. Take a deep breath, relaxing your stomach as your lungs expand.
4. Next, contract your stomach muscles with a quick, sharp movement, exhaling forcefully through your nose.
5. Relax your abdomen, and your inhalation will be passive and automatic.

6. Repeat the forceful expulsion of the breath 5 times in quick succession.

7. When you first try Kapalabhati breathing, you may feel that you are running out of breath. This is natural and occurs because you are not relaxing your abdomen after each exhalation. Slow the frequency of expulsions down so that your inhalation is adequate.

8. Take a few long, deep breaths and do another round, this time increasing to 10 repetitions.

9. If you are comfortable, do a third round and increase the number of expulsions to 15.

10. Sit quietly and breathe normally for a few moments.

If you become dizzy or out of breath, discontinue the exercise and take long, deep breaths. With time and practice you will be able to increase the number of expulsions and the speed with which you do this breath without feeling faint or running out of breath.

Note: Do not practice Kapalabhati during menstruation.

PRANA IN THE AIR

Another aid to mining the moment while on a walk is to pay attention to the energy in the air you breathe. Most of us don't really notice that the air in different spaces has different levels of energy in it. Indoor air simply does not have the same amount of vital energy that outside air does. Since most of our walking takes place outdoors, we have a chance to experience fully the greater life force contained in fresh air. In yogic terms, this energy or life force is referred to as *prana*.

When you begin to pay attention to the energy in the air you breathe, you take one more step away from the preoccupation with your past and dreams of the future, and take one more step into the here and now. To help you absorb more prana into your system, we recommend you practice breathing through your nose as often as you can. In yoga most breathing is done through the nose. Not only do you have a better filtration system in the nose but, according to yogic philosophy, you also have "prana receptors," or organs in the nose for accumulating vital energy from the air for the body and the brain. These prana receptors have the additional role of alerting the other systems in the body that a breath is coming, allowing them to take maximum advantage of the next inhalation. This is the same role our senses of smell and taste play in the digestive process. They alert all parts of the system that a certain type of food is coming so that each organ can do its job to digest the food most completely.

Sensory Awareness of Motion

Usually we walk without paying any attention to the actual motion of our bodies. We're focused on where we are going, not on the sensations of the journey. You can begin to develop sensory awareness by paying attention to the way your body moves through space. When you start to pay attention to the motion of your body, your awareness leads you to a more in-depth experience of the moment. You can feel how each foot strikes the ground and how the walking surface affects the pressure on your ankles, knees, and hips. Just as you do when you focus on the breath, you'll start to experience your walk from the inside out. This experience produces a subtle grounding effect, bringing you home to your body in its most primal physical state.

CROSSLATERAL MOTION

When you start to pay attention to the whole movement of your body, you find the natural rhythm of your arms linking up with the strides of your legs. When we are balanced, the body proceeds with its own integrated knowledge of movement, in which the right arm swings forward in time with the left leg, and vice versa. This crosslateral movement is embedded in the memory banks of our cells. This is the way almost all creatures traverse the earth, and it is a powerful and graceful form of locomotion. When you walk in tune with your primal instincts by using the breath and the crosslateral motion, you access your inherent source of power and grace. You learn to transfer your body's physical strength into grace and fluidity of movement, like that of a cat.

Crosslateral motion is a rhythmic, balanced movement that requires you to relate dynamically to the right and left sides of your body as well as the upper half and the lower half. Research has shown that this movement stimulates both hemispheres and all four lobes of the brain.

The more we are able to access both sides of the brain, the more intelligently we function and the more we can access our emotions and intuition. The reason you feel better emotionally and can think more clearly and creatively at the end of a good long walk is that the crosslateral motion of walking helps build and strengthen the sensory capabilities—auditory, visual, proprioceptive—from both sides of the body. Early childhood research has found that the crosslateral motion of crawling is crucial for activating full sensory functioning and learning in infants. Crawling involves movements that cross the body's midline and engage both sides of the brain in concert. Likewise, when we engage in this type of walk, the coordinated movements of both eyes, both hands, both feet, and the balanced core muscles, activate the brain, improving both sensory awareness and mental capacity.

Are You "Switched Off"?

There are times in life when we can become so overwhelmed that our systems get "switched off." When you are switched off, you lose connection with your natural crosslateral motion and begin to move your arms and legs in a unilateral pattern (arm and leg on the same side moving together), like that of a puppet on a string. This motion occurs when there is a short circuit in the energy signal from the brain to the different systems in the body. When practicing sensory awareness, you may notice yourself falling into this type of movement.

Being switched off can occur when you are worrying about things that could go wrong, or when you are involved in an all-consuming problem or emotional situation. Have you ever found yourself mentally arguing with people who upset you? Our thoughts tend to be circular, repeating the same scenarios, coming to the same conclusions over and over. So much energy is dedicated to thinking, the body's natural movement and coordination gets thrown off.

It is interesting that when the left and right brain get out of sync, thinking becomes separated from speaking. While we may be mentally arguing with someone, our actual ability to communicate diminishes. The key to stopping this obsessive thinking is figuring out how to communicate in the situation. As simple as it sounds, sinking back into the natural rhythms of crosslateral walking can generate a surprising amount of creativity and objectivity. The next time you catch yourself thinking obsessively, try actively focusing on the crosslateral motion as you walk. Let the natural swinging movement connect your thinking with your speech, and the right half of your brain with the left half. Fall back into your most natural self; in that state you can summon the best of your brain to help communicate the most powerful and creative answer to any hurdles you face.

CROSSLATERAL MOTION AND CHAKRA POWER

Crosslateral walking motion also helps you access the power of your physical body. One of the reasons for this connection is that the third chakra is engaged. Also known as the *hara* center in Oriental traditions, the third chakra is located at the navel and coincides with the solar plexus. In the science of yoga, the chakras are centers of energy that form a vertical column in the body and function on both a physical and a more subtle energetic level in the body (see page 137). Each chakra activates and affects the body in a different way. The third chakra relates to power, will, energy, and assertiveness. The element of fire is activated when this chakra is stimulated and generates transformational energy in the body and mind.

Yogis consider the solar plexus the point of connection between an individual being and the intelligent energy of the universe. When you are in the womb, you are fed through the umbilical cord, drawing your life force from your mother into your hara. So this is the place where the universal energy continues to feed you, on an energetic level, after you have separated from your mother. It is considered the area from which life energy emanates. When you walk, imagine that you have golden threads radiating outward from your solar plexus, connecting you with the great web of life and the intelligence that organizes it.

How to walk with third chakra power:

1. Start your walk by taking a moment of stillness and closing your eyes.
2. Plant your feet firmly on the ground. Engage your calf, thigh, buttocks, and abdominal muscles to form a powerful, grounded stance.
3. Lift and extend your torso out of your waist. Stand tall by rolling your shoulders back and down and lengthening your arms all the way through the fingertips.
4. Bring your chin parallel to the ground. Lengthen the back of your neck, and press upward out of the crown of your head.
5. Let your awareness drop into your solar plexus and visualize a reservoir of life force in the core of your body.

6. If you are having trouble connecting to the third chakra, the Kapalabhati breath (see page 102) is an excellent way to reestablish your connection.

7. As you start to walk, connect with that reservoir of energy and let it send energy to the rest of your body like a giant sun warming a solar system.

8. Deepen your breath and oxygenate your system while you let the experience of walking act as a generator of physical and spiritual energy.

9. Even if you are walking in a city, take time to marvel at how the life force can never be denied, how every being is continually striving for full expression despite sometimes overwhelming odds.

10. Allow your walk to inspire a sense of reverence for the natural and boundless world both in and around you.

Practicing the following hatha yoga postures will engage and develop the third chakra by building strength and therefore power in the abdominal area. When the abdomen is strong and toned, the energy in the solar plexus flows more powerfully.

Woodchopper Pose

1. Stand in Mountain pose (see page 59).

2. Place your feet about 2 feet apart.

3. Raise your arms overhead, elbows straight, fingers interlaced, with your spine arched slightly backward.

4. Swing your upper arms, head, and torso down toward the ground, bringing your hands and arms through your legs in one smooth and rapid motion. Forcefully and powerfully exhale the breath with the sound "Ha!"

5. Inhaling, roll back up to a standing position with your arms overhead, then swing down again. Repeat 3 to 5 times.

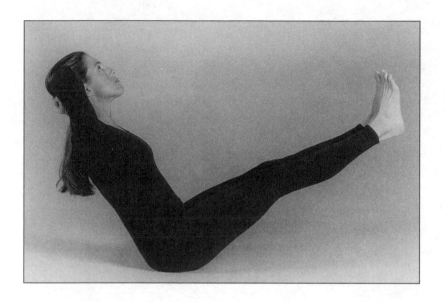

Half Boat Pose

1. Sit with your legs extended in front of you on the mat, heels pushed away and toes flexed toward your body. Feel your buttocks firm against the floor. Place your arms alongside your body, palms on the floor.

2. Inhaling, raise your arms toward the ceiling, extend your spine out of your hips, and extend your head up from your shoulders. Clasp your hands behind your head and point your elbows up toward the ceiling and in toward the body.

3. Lean back, lowering your torso and raising your legs until both are about 30 degrees off the mat. Engage your abdominal muscles to help you balance on your buttocks.

Complete Boat Pose

1. Sit with your legs extended in front of you on the mat, heels pushed away and toes flexed toward your body. Place your arms along-

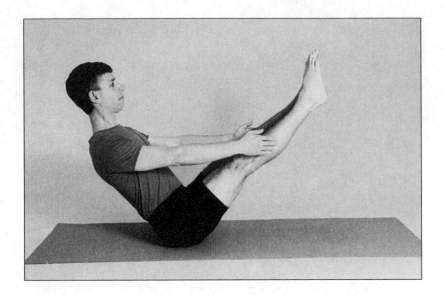

side your body, palms on the floor. Feel your buttocks against the floor.

2. Exhaling, raise both legs off the floor (at approximately a 60-degree angle) and lean your torso back so that you are balancing on your sit bones. Use your hands to help you balance.

3. Elongate your torso by lifting the chest, pressing out of the crown of your head, and looking toward your feet. Do not round your back. Press your lower back in toward your stomach.

4. Straighten your arms from the shoulders toward your knees, keeping your arms parallel to the floor and palms facing each other.

5. Hold this position for as long as you can. Try 10 seconds to start.

POSTURE AND GAIT

Posture and gait are other doorways to awareness of motion. Each of us has a way of moving that is unique. There is a particular way we can hold ourselves and a stride we can take that is perfect for our body size and type. When our posture and gait are balanced and integrated, we can make our movement in space beautiful, effortless, and graceful. When this happens, it generates a feeling of "rightness" in the body. Each one of us has a natural and innate flow of movement that can be relearned and reintegrated.

Our bodies have been shaped by a lifetime of experiences, and each of us has areas of the body that present trouble from time to time. The youthful, supple bodies we have as children give way to older, stiffer bodies. Stress, illness, injury, and emotional trauma all contribute to the aging process and a lifetime's worth of postural deviation. These deviations develop through the neglect of some movements and the overuse of others, usually to compensate for weak muscles or pain. The result is poor posture and reliance on habitual patterns of movement.

When you explore your patterns of movement and investigate the roots of poor posture through practicing sensory awareness, you will in many instances find an interesting correlation between your posture and your thinking habits. You may realize that you jut your chin forward, walking as if life were always a challenge. You may find yourself leaning backward slightly as you walk, as if hesitant to move into new experiences too quickly. A rigid posture can correspond to lack of flexibility in thinking about things in new ways or from other people's point of view. Shoulders hunched up toward the ears can correspond to feeling pressured, with lots of expectations to meet. An unbalanced gait or pain on one side of the body might correspond to an overreliance on one way of getting through life, favoring the analytical over the emotional or vice versa.

When we are born, we move in a completely natural way, and we carry no preconceptions about life and ourselves. Gradually this condition changes as we have experiences, particularly those that are painful or scary. Over time we begin to take on beliefs about the world, other people, and ourselves. These acquired beliefs are a way of protecting ourselves from painful experiences we have had. They function as early warning radar, classifying potential experiences as threats or opportunities before we actually have the experiences themselves. By preclassifying events instead of experiencing them as they are, we try to avoid making the mistakes that led to disappointing experiences in the past. Unfortunately, these preclassifications turn into knee-jerk reactions to unfolding experiences. These reactions, instead of protecting us from repeating the past, tend to lead us into the same ditch over and over again. We misapprehend reality. Our beliefs cause us to magnify imaginary opportunities and minimize very real threats or, conversely, to magnify imaginary risks and minimize very real opportunities. In yogic terms, we lack skillfulness in action (see page 8).

For example, we know a woman who goes from relationship to relationship, always picking guys who will not commit to her and who treat her badly in the end. As a result of being hurt and abandoned so many times, she has come to believe she is unworthy of love and will never find romance. She is extremely afraid of being left alone and unloved, and is constantly vulnerable to the fantasy of eternal romance with the next guy who shows interest in her for a little while. Her knee-jerk reaction is to jump into the relationships immediately, falling for guys without noticing their weaknesses and controlling tendencies. Because of her unconscious belief, she continues to cause the very experience she is trying to avoid.

It's easy to see the effects of unconscious beliefs in other people's lives but not as easy to recognize them in our own. We've all seen people sabotaging good relationships and perpetuating bad ones, taking rash risks in business or staying in jobs that are killing them because they are afraid to leave. We've seen people run from experience to experience, never committing to anything, while others stay stuck within a world too small for them. All these life-constricting behaviors stem from unconscious belief systems. See if you recognize traces of some of the following common negative beliefs in those close to you or yourself:

"You can never trust anyone."
"Those you love will always leave you."
"Always be cautious."
"Life is hard."
"In the end I'll always wind up failing."

Unconscious beliefs control us and rob us of the joy that we felt as children. When beliefs like these fall into your unconscious, you stop noticing that they no longer give an accurate picture of life. Your actual experience is always new and different, but your *interpretation* of your experience gradually becomes habitual, contracted, and closed down to the new. All these beliefs eventually get expressed in the way you move and hold your body. Bringing awareness to your habitual beliefs allows you to choose to keep them or to replace them and move your body in a healthier way.

Practicing sensory awareness (see page 104) with your posture and gait can provide clues to habitual belief systems that you may not be consciously aware of but that are strongly influencing the choices you make. When you start to become aware of these beliefs through your body, you begin to gain control of them in your mind. Becoming conscious of how your life experience has molded and shaped your body is the first step to undoing unhealthy physical and mental patterns.

In order to regain a more erect and graceful posture and a more fluid and free walking gait, engaging in a daily practice of yoga postures is essential. If you have limited time, make sure to practice the Mountain pose (see page 59), Supine Leg Stretch, (see page 49), and one repetition of the Sun Salutation (see page 59) every day.

Walking to Regain Your Youthful Gait and Posture

Prepare for your walk by standing in the Mountain pose, and allowing your life force to flow.

1. Stand with your legs a few feet apart. Lift your right foot off the ground and shake your right leg out. Repeat on the left side.

2. Bring your legs parallel to each other, about 2 feet apart, and plant them firmly on the ground.

3. Draw the strength and power up from the earth into your legs and engage your calf and thigh muscles by pressing the muscles toward the bones.

4. Tuck your tailbone under and push your pubic bone forward. The pelvic girdle becomes level and square so that the hipbones are facing forward like two headlights. Engage your buttocks muscles so that they feel solid and strong.

5. Elongate your waist by lifting your torso out of the waist and hips, lift your sternum, open your chest, and roll your shoulders back and down.

6. Rotate your right hand at the wrist. Then move your right arm in a big circle as if you were doing the backstroke. Next move your right arm in a forward circle, and finally shake out your whole right arm. Repeat with the left arm. Keep your shoulders back and down, and lengthen your arms all the way out through the fingertips.

7. Do three complete rotations of the Neck Roll (see page 45).

8. Lengthen the back of your neck, bring your chin parallel to the ground, and press out of the crown of your head. Your head should float balanced atop your torso and legs.

9. Begin your walk using the crosslateral motion: Your right arm swings forward at the same time as your left leg, as if an internal hinge connects them.

10. As you breathe in, draw energy in through your feet and feel it con-

tinue to travel up through your legs, torso, chest, and head. As you exhale, visualize stiff, frozen muscles relaxing and tension leaving your body through your arms and fingertips. Continue this visualization for at least the first 5 minutes of your walk.

As you walk, let your movements be loose and relaxed; at the same time keep your posture strong and tall.

Integration

When we were watching our fellow pedestrians walk the sidewalks of New York City, we noticed how little attention they paid to their surroundings. We could almost hear them thinking "How soon can I get to where I am going?" Their walk was not an enjoyable, integrated experience but an inconvenience on the way to where they really wanted to be.

The world around us is a vast tapestry of smells, sights, sounds, tastes, and sensations. Walking with wonder at the mystery and complexity of life is a doorway into a personal appreciation of the spiritual side of life. Whether you walk on a city street or a country lane, whether among fall leaves or suburban homes, you are always surrounded by the great spectacle of life. When we talk about turning walking into yoga, we are talking about moving through this world with all your senses fully extended, taking in life to the maximum.

The integrative power of walking yoga can help to reshape both your mind and your body. When you walk, try to walk to the beat of nature's rhythm, listening for the harmony in the song of the universe and attempting to match it. By consciously connecting yourself to the world you are passing through, you start to notice how connected everything else is. You catch glimpses of the magnificent underlying intelligence of nature. You notice how nothing is ever wasted, and how every living thing has a role to play and is in some sort of relationship to all the other living things. Yogis always look to nature to provide clues for living in harmony with themselves and others. We spend so much of our time worrying about how things will work out, but if we watch nature, we can see a larger design and find greater patience.

By bringing conscious breathing practices into your walking, you will find the whole character of your walk changes. Your walk will become an automatic stress reducer. All of your cells get bathed in oxygen, and the stress hormones that accumulate in the bloodstream are eliminated as the blood is systematically cleansed by the breath. You start to notice that during and after your walk you feel more alive and, in a simple way, happier. The combination of walking and practicing deep rhythmic breathing in which you focus on the sound and sensation of the breath can, within a short time, ease the grip that any problem has on your mind and emotions. The circumstances that caused your problem might not have changed, but all of a sudden you feel more optimistic about its resolution. As the breath deepens and your mind quiets, you find that your creativity increases and resolutions to problems appear where none seemed likely before.

Chapter 5

the five ways of walking yoga

Tulips and daffodils bloom on hillsides amid spring rains. Roses and marigolds grace garden paths during long, golden summer days. Chrysanthemums and fiery foliage herald each fall as days grow chill and clouds gather in the west. In the winter snow covers all, while living things rest in their long sleep. Every season plays its role in the mystery of life. Without the cold of winter, the fruit trees will not bear well, and without the summer thunderstorms, the land would be too parched to sustain life.

Each of us also has seasons, moods, and cycles. You are not the same person you were yesterday, and tomorrow you will be different yet again. One day you feel charged up and ready to tackle big projects, and another day or time you want to slow down and reflect. What nurtures you one day may not be the same as what nurtures you another.

True spiritual practice sustains you through all your moods and is flexible enough to adapt to them. Even though everything in nature moves to cycles and rhythms, many of us resist the swings in our moods, energy levels, and circumstances. Part of walking yoga is learning to accept our changing nature and flowing with the change. Sometimes you need to be alone, other times to have company; sometimes you need to walk fast, other times to walk slowly. Use the variety of approaches to walking yoga to adapt to your changing needs.

How Do I Accurately Identify My Body's Needs?

Our society is so fixated on youth and beauty that we often begin to exercise because we feel bad about how we look. There is nothing wrong with getting motivated by vanity, but the problem is that we can subtly use exercise to punish ourselves for being overweight, out of shape, or inflexible. In addition, with this motivation we have no patience for the time it takes to achieve physical results from exercise or a change in our life habits. We've watched many of our students take on yoga and walking with driven determination. They vow to walk three miles every day up the biggest hill they can find. This is fine for the first two weeks, but what then? Six months later these people have given up walking. It's impossible to sustain a practice when it comes from a place of force and coercion, even if that coercion is self-induced.

Rigidity in practice leads to injury and frustration, and both of these lead to failure and quitting. The sixth-century B.C.E. Chinese sage and poet Lao-tzu wrote that rigidity and hardness are signs of aging and death, whereas flexibility and softness are characteristics of youth and life. We have found that the best approach to a sustained walking yoga practice is to approach your walks from a place of loving yourself and your body by gently coaxing and inspiring yourself to better health and vitality. You must develop patience and an ability to respond to your personal needs and circumstances. How can you do this reliably? Trust yourself and listen. Listen inside to what you need, and listen outside to what is present for you to connect to.

THE OVERACHIEVER: IGNORING THE BODY'S NEEDS

When Carol started her walking yoga practice, she was determined to get that ideal body she had always dreamed of. She had read about the muscle-sculpting effects of yoga in an article in *Time* magazine. Since our workshop also offered walking, she thought adding walking to the mix would speed things up for her. Carol had a strong competitive drive, which made her successful in business but less successful with her health and love life. She was very proud of her success as a partner in a law firm in New York City, but she felt she had neglected her body and was overweight and out of shape. Carol was thirty-five and not yet married, and in her mind time was running out. She had an image of what she should look like to attract a potential husband, and she was determined to achieve it. In addition, she wanted to sustain her health so that she could keep up with the rigorous schedule required of a partner in a law firm.

Whenever we went on walks during the first few days of the workshop, Carol was way out in front, arms swinging, hips churning, breath puffing, determined to burn away calories and slim her ample hips. During the yoga sessions Carol would push herself beyond her capacity to work her muscles harder and stay at the head of the class. Carol was approaching the class as she had always approached her life. Her belief that you have to work hard and push to exhaustion to be successful was a long-held habit. On the third day of the class Carol was so sore and exhausted that she could hardly move.

We talked about what was going on for Carol and helped her to consider that she could achieve her goal of a toned, strong, and energized body in a much more caring way. She started to see that following her own rhythms and needs would allow her to accomplish her goals in a way that integrated her more aggressive and disciplined self with her slower, more nurturing self. There are times when it's appropriate to push and challenge, but these need to be integrated with who you are and the condition of your body. Carol began to see that slow and gentle efforts were equally important in building a strong and healthy body. True strength is both strong and flexible, firm yet pliable. Carol didn't lose as much weight or build as much muscle as she had imagined she would in her week with us, but she has a new lifestyle that she loves and has been able to sustain over time. Her walking yoga practice has become a path for generating a healthy and balanced life instead of the quick fix she came looking for.

THE UNDERACHIEVER: IGNORING THE BODY'S NEEDS

Most of us are afraid to listen to our bodies' needs because we fear we would end up staying in bed all day. Laziness, avoidance, and lack of discipline can be as detrimental to the body as pushing it too hard. The overachiever and the underachiever are two sides of the same coin. Our student Jennifer shared this story with us about her struggles with self-discipline.

"I had a gifted mind, excelled at school, and generally succeeded at whatever I did. At a critical period of uncertainty and soul-searching in my life, I was faced with the need to take care of my body. I began a yoga practice, and that's when I found the underachiever, the one who couldn't quite commit.

"Despite the energy and confidence my yoga practice brought me, I resisted it. I continued to smoke yet another cigarette, sometimes just after practice. I skipped class and cluttered up the space I had created for practicing yoga at home. I would move in and out of being more committed and breaking my commitments. It's not that I felt I didn't have enough time in life. In fact, I felt that I had all the time in the world, so why do it now?

"Bringing the awareness I was learning in the yoga postures on my walks, I was able to come into a deeper understanding of just how I put things off, and how bad I felt mistreating my body. Deep down, I was waiting for someone else to take care of my body for me. Including other people in my commitment to walking yoga helped make regular practice more enjoyable. I walked with one friend three times a week and checked in with another friend daily (she was learning sitting meditation). Inspiring thoughts began to outweigh resistant thoughts, feeling good in my body began to satisfy me more than smoking cigarettes.

"I started to transfer more and more of the positive yoga experience to other parts of my life. I would flake out sometimes and backslide with my practice, but it was a little less each time. I think the most important thing that I learned from this practice is to respect the natural desires of my body. My overachieving earlier in life was always to please someone else. My underachieving came from not focusing on pleasing myself. As I come more and more into balance, I find willpower and self-motivation generating from the inside. Sometimes when I least expect it, I'll find myself getting up from my desk and stretching into a yoga pose, wondering how I got there."

Accurately identifying your body's needs—being able to distinguish when you need a more rigorous workout with a buddy from when you need a more contemplative walk by yourself—comes with experience. In the beginning, though, when you resist the thought of a walk and your body is craving chocolate or caffeine, you can assume it really needs to be receiving more oxygen and to get your blood pumping. Your body needs some form of physical exercise every day because regular practice is the only way to reset the body's learned and habituated patterns so that your natural urges become powerful enough for you to hear.

You will learn more tips for accurately identifying your body's needs and maintaining a regular practice in Chapter 7. For now, when you start to incorporate walking yoga into your life, do it gently. Be creative, and let every walk be as different as you are each time you walk. Your love for yourself, your walk, and your world will always show you a way to connect to the beauty and spirit of each walk.

The Five Ways of Walking Yoga

While every walk is different, we have discovered in our own practice that there are some recurring themes amid the nuances and shadings that make each walk unique. These themes act as doorways to the yoga of the walk, ways to drop into the center of the present moment, where ordinary locomotion becomes walking yoga. We will treat them as different ways of walking, each an invitation to meld with a different sort of personal tone or timbre that suits the changing warp and woof of the unfolding tapestry of your life.

FULL-ON-WALKING

The yoga of full-on-walking is to be totally within your body at its peak of exertion. In this walk you fall into that zone where you are filled with sensation and are beyond thinking.

We like to practice full-on-walking after days when everything feels like it's coming apart at work. You know, the days when people have let us down, held us up, missed the point, or otherwise obstructed our idea of how the day should unfold. When we get home and find ourselves still carrying on unfinished conversations, we know that full-on-walking is a reliable antidote to banish the crowd from our heads and the stress from our blood. We lace up our shoes and do a few warm-up stretches, then stride out the door to climb the hill that runs for a mile near our house. It's very difficult to continue those one-sided, disembodied arguments when our hearts are laboring just to supply our bodies with enough oxygen to keep going forward.

When you practice full-on-walking, you are sidling down the continuum toward the animal side of you. The exertion dictates your focus. The body becomes primary, the mind, secondary. Instead of chewing over things that went wrong during the day or possible disasters lurking around the corner, you are filled with the sensations of physical living. Whether you're climbing a hill or moving on the flat, your arms are swinging, your breath is hard, and your steps are long and rapid. You feel the walk draw you into itself, absorbing you in the moment. The effort demands being fully present with the physical sensory experience: breath blowing like a bellows; sweat streaming from your pores, releasing toxins; and heat radiating off your skin, creating a glow all over your body. Full-on-walking induces that state Thoreau described when he wrote, "The whole body is one sense, and imbibes delight through every pore."

The benefits of full-on-walking long outlast your walk by providing the stamina required to deal with whatever life brings your way. There are times when we are challenged to our mental and emotional limit, and we have to perform with our maximum capacity in order to survive and succeed. The benefits that come from training your body and mind to function at their peak levels of exertion will aid you greatly in such times of need. In addition, full-on-walking develops the third chakra and its associated functions of willpower, drive, and focus. These powerful tools are further resources when we are in need of inner strength.

Getting Started with Full-on-Walking

Warm up the body with a series of yoga postures chosen from Chapter 3. For a simple routine, include the Butterfly, Knee Down Twist, Forward Bend, and one Sun Salutation. If you are short of time, simply stand on a curb with your heels hanging over for a few minutes to stretch out your calf muscles and do three Neck Rolls.

If you want to do a more elaborate yoga routine before you start, make sure to include the Supine Leg Stretch, Butterfly, Forearm Stretch, Cobra, Forward Bend, and at least two rounds of the Sun Salutation. These basic postures will ensure that your muscles are limber and warm for your walk.

Before you start walking, bring your attention to your standing posture. Be sure to stand straight and tall, lift out of your waist, raise your sternum, roll your shoulders back and down, lengthen your arms by your sides and out through the fingertips, and press up through the crown of your head. These adjustments give you a sense of what equilibrium feels like in your body and will help align and balance your movement, reducing the chance of injury.

In this standing posture, with your eyes open, begin practicing the complete yogic breath with Ujjayi breathing for 2 to 3 minutes (see pages 98 and 101). The rhythm and sound of the breath will help to calm your mind and prepare your body for the more intense aerobic workout of full-on-walking. You are now ready to start your walk with the crosslateral motion, swinging the right arm forward in time with the left leg stepping out and vice versa. Find a walking rhythm that feels comfortable and fluid. If possible, start walking on level ground and take 5 to 10 minutes for warm-up walking. In this warm-up period, and in the cooldown, breathe through your nose if possible.

Coordinate your breath with the number of steps that are most comfortable for you to take. On level ground, aim to take at least four steps for every inhalation and four steps for every exhalation. Ujjayi breathing helps you to moderate this rhythm. You want your breath to be long and deep, filling the lungs completely on the inhalation, then emptying them thoroughly on the exhalation. You'll notice that as you synchronize your breath with the steps, you'll naturally start to walk faster, and you'll feel power seeping into your muscles. You can always adjust the number of steps you take per breath according to your exertion and depending on the slope of the hill. The steeper the incline, the fewer steps you can take with each breath. The important point is to establish a walking-breathing rhythm and regulate it as needed.

Bringing Awareness to Your Third Chakra

Once you have established a comfortable walking and breathing rhythm, move your focus to your solar plexus or third chakra (see page 106). Engage the abdominal muscles slightly and allow your strength to come from the center of your body. You may find when you time your breath to your steps that your awareness automatically moves to the third chakra. That's because it is the center of power in the body and gives you access to power in life. From a consistent practice of full-on-walking, in which the third chakra is engaged, you will gain a sense of mastery in both body and mind. The more you practice, the more you will develop a kinesthetic, or body memory of core strength, which then becomes available to you in other aspects of your life.

Focusing on the third chakra, gradually begin to pick up the pace and/or increase the slope of your walk. At this point you want to elevate the heart rate and breathing so that you are fully engaged in the experience and your mind is forced to pay attention to what you are doing.

This experience is always uplifting because your body is being pumped full of health-producing endorphins and you sweat out the excess stress hormones you collected during the day or the previous day. Full-on-walking is like taking a shower on the inside of your body. The increased velocity and volume of your circulatory and lymphatic systems, along with the increased volume and velocity of the breath, scrub the transport channels in your body, bringing oxygen and nutrients to each cell and carrying away carbon dioxide and metabolic wastes. When you change your biochemistry, you also change your mood and outlook. We find that full-on-walking hardly ever fails to renew our optimism and recharge our batteries. Sometimes we come back from a full-on-walk elated, even though we started out cranky and upset.

Once you reach your peak, try to keep this pace for at least 15 minutes (longer if you can). For the most part, your attention will be on the breath and the sensation of effort in your body. Once you are at peak effort you'll find that the Ujjayi breath becomes difficult, and you'll naturally stop doing it. Allow your breath to transition to a natural, heavy pattern suited to high exertion.

Full-on-walking produces the most direct aerobic health benefits of any kind of walking and should be practiced as often as the spirit moves you to do so. Aerobic exercise is a form of exercise that uses large muscles rhythmically and continuously and elevates the heart rate and breathing for a sustained period of time. Most experts agree that aerobic exercise should be done at least three times a week for 20 minutes or longer. Aerobic exercise is a key component of long-term vitality in life, and its benefits have been communicated effectively through the media. If you want more precise information on aerobic exercise, refer to *The Aerobics Program for Total Well-Being* by Kenneth Cooper, M.D.

Tips for walking at your peak:

- If you are not sure of your cardiovascular health, start slowly and monitor your effort closely. It's better to build up your endurance over time rather than try to max out the first time. Taking things gradually is especially important if you are out of shape, overweight, or recovering from an illness or injury.

- You should be able to talk comfortably while you are exercising, even if you choose not to. If you're breathing too hard to talk, you're probably overdoing it.

- Trust your perception of how hard your workout is. Don't get caught up in thinking you should be keeping up with someone when you are struggling.

- After your warm-up period, you want to sustain your aerobic level and break a sweat for at least 12 to 15 minutes of your walk. Keep moving to cool down for 10 minutes after.

We recommend practicing full-on-walking at least three or four times a week, for 45 minutes each time, including warm-up and cooldown. On most weekends we walk for three hours or more. You can extend your own full-on-walking practice over time.

WALKING ALONE

I never found the companion that was as companionable as solitude.—*Henry David Thoreau*

Walking alone can be a time to sort things out, mull things over, meander, explore, and strike that subtle balance between being and doing. It's a time to find yourself by giving the body, mind, and spirit an opportunity to align as well as interact, as if three good friends were in dialogue. And, perhaps most important, walking alone can provide so much solace for the soul that some people compare it to attending church. It is a time to sort through our greatest troubles, worries, and fears and face life on our own.

There is a verse from a traditional gospel song, popularized by Woody Guthrie and Elvis Presley, that states.

> *You've got to walk*
> *that lonesome valley*
> *Walk it yourself*
> *You've gotta gotta go*
> *by yourself*
> *Ain't nobody else*
> *gonna go there for you*
> *Yea, you've gotta go*
> *there by yourself.*

There are times when we have to face things on our own. We go through life fearing and resisting being alone when in reality true power and happiness can come only from a cellular comfort with our own aloneness. It's a paradox that owning your fundamental separateness is the doorway to true connection and union. How can this be? Our fear of being alone stems from looking to get our needs met outside ourselves, seeking approval, acceptance, security, and self-esteem from other people. Usually we live in a world of fantasy regarding the people around us, imagining motives, connections, and contracts that do not exist. We often assume that others will fulfill our personal needs and that we are more important pieces of their lives than we actually are. As a result, they continually throw us off, dashing our hidden expectations and fantasies. Other people often disappoint us, but we don't usually recognize that our disappointment is caused as much by our expectation of them as it is by their behavior. Many times we don't even know we have these unspoken contracts and fantasies until they go unfulfilled and we are left with the roil of anger and hurt surging in our bellies.

Walking Alone Gives Insight

For the first time in nearly twenty years the Kripalu Yoga Fellowship was going to choose a new chief executive officer, who would steward the work, values, and mission of the fellowship, which served as the yogic path and spiritual focus for thousands of people.

I was one of two nominees for the post. I had been on the board since its inception nearly fifteen years before. I was a member of the monastic community and had devoted the last eighteen years of my life to the study and practice of a yogic lifestyle. I wanted to be the CEO. I had worked for my entire adult life in the organization, and much of its success and growth bore the imprint of my ideas and leadership. I felt I had earned the right to lead by demonstrating leadership. I assumed my co-workers and board members would see the value of my contribution.

The vote was preceded by a discussion, and my insides began to twist as I saw things were not to go smoothly. I realized the room contained many years of history and unexpressed feelings about the community as a whole. I was a symbol of the old, and people wanted a change. My heart sank as I listened to the discussion about who would be most suitable for CEO. I began to feel a tremendous amount of pain and rejection.

I can still recall people's faces as the votes built up against me. These people I loved so much looked at me like a stranger. My hurt and anger at them coursed through my

continued on next page

mind and my body as I left the meeting in a red fog of confusion.

That night I walked alone. In the measured sound of my footfalls echoing on the street, I came face-to-face with my Self. Who must I have been to be treated like this? What were they seeing in me that I didn't see in myself? What were the ways I behaved that would have caused these people to choose another to lead them? As the earth went by beneath my feet, I walked into uncharted land in my own consciousness. My unconscious habits, ambitions, fears, hopes, dreams, and fantasies were suddenly laid bare, invisible no longer. I saw myself through the board's eyes, and found truth in their sight.

Rather than feeling smaller by seeing my warts and failings, I felt empowered. They might be warts, but they were there because of me, and no other. The anger and betrayal left me, and I felt for the first time that I truly owned the course of my life. I was alone, but being so left me free.

I now regard that fateful day as the most important of my life. From that day forward I was able to understand how I appeared to other people in my worst moments. I gained control of my unconscious and off-putting compensation mechanisms by seeing them as others saw them. Most important, I discovered that I could feel in my body what it was like to be thrown into my insecurity-driven behavior. It was no longer invisible to me.

From that time forward I never cared for others' approval in the same way. Thrown back on my own resources, I discovered that I was enough as I was, beyond anybody else's opinion.

Garrett

Yoga's essence lies in seeing things as they are, without expectation, fantasy, or fear. There is a Zen saying: "When a child looks at a mountain, he sees a mountain; when an adult looks at a mountain, he sees many things, such as a place for recreation, valued real estate, or a mining opportunity; when a sage looks at a mountain, he sees a mountain." We spend so much energy resisting discomfort or pain and chasing after pleasure that we no longer enjoy experiencing life as it is. Walking alone can help you face your life. When you see your life as it truly is, you have real power, because in truth only you have the power to change your life. When you can change your life, others have very little power over you.

Our friend Anne is a poignant example of coming to terms with the fear of being alone and learning to take control of your life. Anne's husband of ten years was a drug addict who would get sober every few months for a few months but then would get caught up with drugs again. Even though she thought she should leave, Anne had two young girls and couldn't imagine raising them on her own. After many years of hoping, praying, and fantasizing that her husband would get better, she finally faced the fact that he never would.

When Anne really analyzed what kept her in the fantasy that her husband would change, that he would get better and they would lead a normal life together, she found her fear of being alone. It was a deeply ingrained fear that she'd developed in childhood in a family setting where she was neglected and emotionally abused. When she looked honestly at herself, she realized she wanted someone to take care of her. As a child, she would dream of having loving parents who nurtured her and cared for her. As an adult, she dreamed of being married to a reliable and caring man who would be a strong father figure for her daughters and a good provider. Anne was unconsciously choosing to be in a marriage with an absentee father and husband, re-creating her unhappy childhood, rather than face her life alone with no one to care for her.

In addition to therapy, practicing walking yoga alone on a regular basis helped Anne face her fear of being alone and learn to believe in herself. The time she spent on her walks helped her begin to cherish the idea of being on her own. She began to feel freedom and inner strength. Walking alone helped her learn to rely on herself in a way she had never experienced.

Most of us have a hard time with our relationships in part because we don't spend enough time alone. It's hard to know where you end and the other begins if you never spend time with yourself. Most of us look for nurturance from activities and people outside of us. When we feel needy, sad, or frantic, we run to our old friends for that soothing sense of having a place in the world. Sometimes these old friends are people we can relax with, and other times they are life habits we grow to depend on. We pour the drink, eat the ice cream, smoke the joint, or watch the television movie as a way to relax. Sometimes we do all these things at once, combining our habits to pump up the volume of the experience. When we get time with no one else around, we fill the space with entertainment, so we aren't really alone even then. Most of us are uncomfortable being alone for very long without a radio, television, computer, stereo, or book engaging us in some way.

Walking alone and silently provides the ideal way to spend time with yourself. When you walk alone, you have a chance to stand on your own two feet, and your pace divides the silence into a quiet rhythm. You'll start to hear the subtle rhythms and textures of nature, both outside and inside of you. You don't have to worry very much about being interrupted, and your walk allows you time to reflect on your problems, giving you additional perspective. While walking in silence you can actively tune in to your own intuition and inner guidance. You'll be amazed at how reliably an answer to a knotty and confusing problem will float to the surface from deep inside when given the chance. You have a fountain of wisdom right inside you; all you need to do is take the time to listen.

When you walk alone your biochemistry joins in providing you a chance for clear thinking. Your deep breath brings oxygen to your cells, and the walk stimulates your system to metabolize stress hormones and expel toxins. As your blood cleans up, you think more clearly, and see more truly. The brain is stimulated by the coordinated movements of both sides of the body, helping you to think more creatively. The overall experience is one of integration and peace.

Silent Rhythms

I used to sit on the bulkhead at the end of our street and watch my mother walk off down the endless stretch of beach that was our front yard. She would always walk alone, often in bare feet, letting the ocean waves wash over her and carry away the countless hidden burdens that only a mother could know. She looked beautiful silhouetted against the vast stretch of blue, drenched in sunlight. As a child, I wondered why she walked alone. As an adult, I learned of her struggle with raising six children, the loss of a child, and the ups and downs in her marriage. Walking alone became her sanctuary, confessional, and source of renewal. The rhythm of her walking generated a rhythm to her thinking, allowing her to clear her mind, face her fears, and sort through the rich soil of her emotions. Being in silence and listening to the rhythmic sound of the ocean waves gave her a feeling of being encapsu-

continued on next page

lated in a womb. She would always return with a smile and an almost ethereal look on her face, as if she had been with an old and beloved friend.

Ila

A Practice for Walking Alone

Before you start your walk, take 10 to 15 minutes to stretch your body with a few Neck Rolls, one repetition of the Sun Salutation, the Tree pose (for balance), Yoga Mudra, and the Forward Bend, as described in Chapter 3. Also include a few minutes of Kapalabhati and Ujjayi breathing, as described in Chapter 4, after performing the postures. You want to center yourself and begin the process of introversion or connecting inside.

If possible pick a place to walk in a natural setting, with trees, grass, water, and/or open sky. It's helpful if the environment feels nurturing, safe, and beautiful to you. Stand for a moment at the beginning of the path or road you plan to walk and notice how your feet are connected to the earth, your body rising straight up from the ground, perfectly balanced and tall, connecting to the sky.

Begin your walk using the crosslateral motion. Swing your right leg forward, stepping on your heel; roll forward onto the ball of the foot; balance on the ball and toes of the right foot, and push off the big toe of your left foot as you swing your left leg forward. Your right arm swings forward at the same time as the left leg, as if an internal hinge connects them. Walk at a natural pace.

Breathe deeply, using the Ujjayi breath (see page 101), and start by counting the steps you take with every inhalation and every exhalation. This counting will help you focus on the present moment. Try to set aside at least 30 to 45 minutes for this walk so you won't feel rushed, and you will be able to sink into the experience.

Visualize each step turning the wheel of your life forward, with you at its center. As your body moves, watch your thoughts circle in the usual way for a while and then start to question their potency. See if you can look the problem square in the face and search out the part you played in its development. Let each step move you further from the fantasy of magical deliverance and closer to a clear acceptance of the reality. When you walk alone, you can see your thoughts more clearly, which helps you take responsibility for your situation. You move from "I wish" and "if only" to "I can."

As you walk, allow each step to become a symbol for you being "at cause" in your own life. In other words, nothing that happens to you happens without you. As you practice, you will start to see how your desires, fears, and expectations played a role in landing you in any difficulties you face, and that you have the power to change them. You can reduce your desires if they are creating pain for you. You can face your fears when you see how they cause trouble. You can manage your expectations when they lead you to be hurt. You can master your addictions if they are destroying your health and relationships. None of these changes is easy, but they can be achieved one step at a time.

For the last 10 to 15 minutes of your walk, move into silence both internally and externally. Start to listen for the answers to your questions and the solutions to your problems. Listen to your inner wisdom and find comfort in your own company. When you get home, take a minute to write down one or two realizations, inspirations, or ideas that came from this time alone.

Adding a Mantra

Repeating a sound or a mantra while you walk alone can be a powerful tool for calming the mind and sending good vibrations through your whole body, helping to reduce stress and enhance your overall sense of well-being. The sound vibrations of mantras have the capacity to improve spatial perception and mental and verbal communication. The Sanskrit word *mantra* means "instrument of thought."

You can repeat the mantra out loud, hum it to yourself, or repeat it silently in your head depending on your comfort level and circumstances. Here are a few suggestions of mantras you may want to try:

- Ila's mother likes to chant the well-known Buddhist mantra *Aum Mane Padme Hum* (pronounced "om mahnee pahdmay hum") during her walks. It has a soothing, relaxing feeling to it and can be loosely translated as "the jewel in the lotus."

- *Shri Ram, Jai Ram, Jai, Jai, Ram* (pronounced "shree rom jai rom jai jai rom," *jai* rhymes with *I*) is one of the Sanskrit chants more commonly sung in the West. This easy, melodic chant has an uplifting effect and can be repeated over and over to the pace of your walk. In one of the great sagas of Indian mythology, the Ramayana, the story of the legendary and heroic lord Rama, unfolds. This mantra, roughly translated, means "Victory to Lord Ram, whose characteristics embody those of the life-sustaining force in nature." In essence the mantra is used to bring joy and gratitude into your heart for the elements in life that feed and sustain you.

- *Om Namah Shivaya* (pronounced "om nahmah sheevieya") is another powerful mantra that is helpful to chant, especially when you are in a period of change and transformation. In Hinduism, Shiva is the aspect of the Divine that represents transformation. Roughly translated, this mantra means "I bow to Shiva" and is chanted as an appeal to God to help us change those things we find almost impossible to alter ourselves.

If you would like to listen to mantras being chanted, write Spring Hill Music, Box 800, Boulder, CO 80306, or phone them at 303-938-

1188 to get a catalog of mantra-chanting CDs. You can also order many mantra-chanting tapes from Amazon.com.

There are also specific mantras you can use to stimulate a particular chakra, or energy center, in the body. The chakra system is inextricably linked with the science of yoga and represents the intersection where mind, body, and spirit meet. There are seven chakras, which form a vertical column, each located near one of the seven major nerve ganglia that emanate from the spinal column. Each chakra has a characteristic quality, such as survival, desire, willpower, love, communication, clarity, and wisdom, as well as corresponding attributes such as sound vibrations, glands, colors, emotions, and insights. Using the seed sound, or mantra, that correlates to a specific chakra while you walk strengthens that power center. When chanting the mantra, take a deep breath in and say the mantra on the exhalation, drawing out the final *m* sound as long as your exhalation lasts, as if you were humming it. Here are examples of mantras that stimulate the chakras:

First Chakra: Also known as the *Muladhara* or root chakra, the first chakra is located at the perineum near the base of the spine and is associated with our basic survival needs, health, comfort, and security. *Lam* (rhymes with *Tom*) is the seed sound used to stimulate this chakra and is a good mantra to chant when you are feeling ungrounded, insecure, or afraid, or if you are experiencing sciatica, exhaustion, intestinal problems, or weakness in the bones or skeleton. Chanting this mantra can nourish your root energy and increase your stability and groundedness, and your sense of safety in life. As you walk, chant the sound *Lam* and visualize a warm, ruby red circle of light surrounding the base of your spine.

Second Chakra: The second chakra, also known as the *Swadhisthana* chakra, is located in the lower abdomen, centered between the genitals and the navel. The second chakra is associated with movement and flow, emotion, nurturance, pleasure, and sexuality. *Vam* (rhymes with

Tom) is the seed sound used to stimulate this chakra and is a good mantra to chant when you are preparing to conceive; dealing with infertility, impotence, or decreased sex drive; or experiencing bladder or kidney trouble. Chanting this mantra can increase your sense of fluidity, passion, and emotional balance. As you walk, chant the sound *Vam* and visualize a warm orange circle of light surrounding your womb, genitals, and lower abdomen.

Third Chakra: The third chakra, also known as the *Manipura* chakra, is located between the navel and the solar plexus and helps strengthen your will, power, and sense of assertiveness. It is helpful to repeat the mantra *Ram* (rhymes with *Tom*) in tune with your walking when you are feeling powerless and angry or if you are dealing with digestive disorders. As you walk, focus your attention on your solar plexus, visualize a warm yellow light growing in your abdominal region, and allow the sound vibration of *Ram* to stimulate the energy vortex in this region of your body.

Fourth Chakra: The fourth chakra, also known as the *Anahata* chakra, is located at the heart and is associated with love, relationship, healing, and unity. *Yam* (rhymes with *Tom*) is the seed sound used to stimulate this chakra and is a good mantra to chant when you are dealing with grief and a broken heart or if you are experiencing asthma, heart problems, or lung disease. Chanting this mantra can open your heart, improve your capacity to love, and rejuvenate your sense of self-acceptance. As you walk, chant the sound *Yam* and visualize a warm, emerald green circle of light surrounding your heart.

Fifth Chakra: The fifth chakra, also known as the *Vissudha* chakra, is located at the throat and is associated with communication and creativity. The seed sound used to stimulate this chakra is *Ham* (rhymes with *Tom*). It is a good mantra to chant to help strengthen your power and courage in communicating what you think and feel, or if you have thyroid problems, hearing problems, a sore throat or a cold. As you walk, chant the sound *Ham* and visualize a circle of bright blue light in the center of your throat.

Sixth Chakra: Aum, or *Om,* is considered the most powerful mantra in the chakra system and is associated with the sixth chakra, also known as the *Ajna* chakra. The sixth chakra is located between the eyebrows in what is referred to as the third eye center. This center corresponds to the pineal gland and is considered the command center of the body. While you walk, repeat the sound of *Om* and visualize a warm circle of indigo light and energy developing in the center of your forehead. This will strengthen your general sense of energy, light, and luminescence in the body and increase your power of imagination. Use this mantra if you are experiencing headaches, eye problems, or nightmares.

Seventh Chakra: The seventh or crown chakra's Sanskrit name is *Sahasrara,* which means "thousandfold," and this chakra is often referred to as the thousand-petaled lotus. The seventh chakra is located at the top of the head and represents consciousness, which is experienced through the element of thought. This center corresponds to the pituitary gland and in yogic philosophy is considered the seat of enlightenment. There is no specific seed sound that corresponds to this chakra, but the function of the *Sahasrara* is knowing and complete awareness. The seventh chakra relates to the cerebral cortex and the nervous system on a physiological level and acts as a meeting place between the earthly and the divine. Development of the seventh chakra is done through the practice of meditation. Use the exercises described in contemplative walking (see page 153) to practice walking meditation and focus your awareness on the crown chakra. Visualize a violet or white light surrounding the top of your head, particularly if you are feeling depressed, confused, or disenchanted.

Adding an Affirmation

An affirmation is a short phrase you can repeat when you want to develop strength and power within yourself and, in a sense, reprogram some of the negative beliefs you have picked up over the course of your life. One example of an affirmation is "I am strong, healthy, capable, and complete within myself." Repeating this over and over to yourself begins to train your mind to think and eventually act differently. You can make up an affirmation that is perfectly suited to your life and circumstance. When you do, be sure it is in the positive present; use "I am" instead of "I will." For example, "I am confident and fearless," instead of "I will let go of my fears."

WALKING WITH LOVED ONES

As much as we need time alone and in silence, we also need intimacy and connection. There is perhaps no goal more sought after by humans than true intimacy with another human. Like a compass needle, which always swings to north, each of us is always yearning to be more connected to the people around us. Being truly known by someone renders us more whole in a way that is difficult to reach by ourselves. We lack this wholeness because we are often cut off from the richness of our own emotions. We find ourselves bedeviled by the churn and roil of our deeper feelings. Anger, shame, insecurity, jealousy, sexuality, and petty selfishness play hide-and-seek with the veneer of social acceptability we show to the world.

Mostly we keep our inner worlds locked away. Few people know the faces of their primal selves, the ones that idly imagine romantic fantasy, are full of pride, plot retaliation, experience hurts, disappointments, and outrage. In most cases this is as it should be. Seldom does life call for such deep self-revealing. Unfortunately, in keeping this world completely secret, we risk losing touch with it ourselves. When we lose touch with these primitive urges and motivations, they don't go away. They become unconscious and lie in wait for a chance to express themselves—usually with unfortunate results.

Garrett remembers, "Many years ago, I was the executive director of Kripalu ashram during a time when it was expanding rapidly and I was taking on more and more responsibility. I felt quite burdened by the increasing stress in my job. One day the founder of the ashram, Yogi Amrit Desai, and Krishnapriya, the CEO, were traveling to India, and I was to drive them to the airport so we could talk business during the trip. I knew I had been feeling invisible and unappreciated for my work, but I would always push those feelings aside as unworthy of attention and 'unspiritual.' My feelings of resentment never even registered on my radar screen.

"Of course, we were late leaving, and everyone was rushing around trying to get going. I took the suitcases to the back of the big Buick we were driving to the airport, and everyone piled in.

"I strapped on my seat belt, checked the mirrors, and put the car into reverse. As the Buick accelerated, the right rear of the car rolled up and over some unknown object. It felt as if I had run over a small boulder even though I knew there was no rock in the driveway. Shocked and disoriented by the sudden lurch, I immediately put the car back into drive so I could reverse my position and get away from the obstacle. Again the back tire lifted off the ground and rolled over a fairly large object. Everyone jumped from the car to see what had happened.

"One of the suitcases, a brand-new Samsonite, lay on the ground, crushed and mutilated, with two neatly defined tire tracks ground into its cover, one from backing up, the other the return trip. Worse, Amrit loved avocados and had packed a supply in the suitcase. When we finally got the suitcase open, the clothes were stained avocado green and Amrit had to pack a whole new suitcase. We did manage to get things sorted out and make the plane, but I was mortified and Amrit and Krishnapriya were pretty upset. How had I forgotten to put the suitcase in the trunk?

"At first, it seemed like a simple case of forgetting the suitcase in the rush of the moment. But when I thought more about it, I came to realize that forgetting was an act of aggression against Amrit and Krishnapriya, because deep inside I felt taken advantage of and unappreciated. As I related the incident to my co-workers amidst gales of laughter, I realized I was partly gleeful at the destruction I had caused. By losing touch with what I really felt, I had to deal with a much messier situation (in more ways than one) than if I had dealt with my feelings directly."

Being intimate means risking giving a voice to some of that netherworld of the beast inside us. This revelation is always difficult, scary, and fraught with risk. When we tell our deeper feelings and emotions to another, we take the chance that the person will run away from such honesty, or judge us for having such base motivations and selfish perspectives.

Avoiding these risks is not free however. When you hide your true feelings, you can't really explain your behavior, either to yourself or to your loved one. Your explanations are at odds with your actions, and you leave your loved one puzzled and confused. Sometimes people experience unexpected bursts of anger, going into a towering rage over a seemingly small event. Losing touch with small resentments and dissatisfactions inevitably leads to indirect expressions of those feelings over irrelevant issues. Such misdirection complicates relationships because you wind up talking about the wrong issues. It also undermines trust.

Once mistrust is present, each partner starts to misconstrue the other's behavior, ascribing motives and purposes to supply an explanation for otherwise bewildering actions. "He must watch television because he doesn't care about how I feel," or "She must be trying to keep me from watching sports because she always needs to control everything." Accusations fly from these misapprehensions, and defenses rise from the sense of unfair indictment. Both people end up feeling hurt, angry, and misunderstood. Distance grows, hiding increases, and love withers.

Taking time to communicate across these misunderstandings and hurt feelings is critical, and walking together is an ideal way to do this. One of the big blocks to getting at the deeper issues is time. You say, "We just can't set aside enough uninterrupted time to talk it all out. The phone rings, the kids scream, the chores beckon." When you walk, you are free from interruptions and distractions. No one else is there. Plan a long walk, and you know you are in for two or three hours of focused time.

Uninterrupted time together is likely to deliver results for another reason as well. Because most of our deeper feelings skirt the edges of conscious awareness, access to them is often defended psychologically. We don't tell our secrets willingly or easily. At the beginning of a conversation, we make a quick, unconscious assessment of the time allotted for the talk and arrive at an unspoken decision on how deep we can go. If the time is too short, we never go deep enough. When you are out on a long walk, it's easier to broach the defenses.

Beyond time, the very act of walking brings to the surface that which lies between you. Each step is like the stroke of a butter churn, working the cream to the surface. Unfinished business floats to the top when you are with someone you love, giving you a chance to clear up incomplete communications. As you walk, each step moves the body toward a higher level of functioning. The blood moves more quickly, the lymph system carries away waste, the sweat glands excrete toxins, and the breath releases cellular poisons and floods your cells with oxygen. The fluid movement of your walking helps to create the ideal physical, mental, and emotional conditions for communicating.

Tender or scary communications need the right pacing, and the pace of the walk yields a rhythm for the gradual unfolding of the story. Sometimes you need to walk in silence to digest what has been said during your talk with your loved one and to sort out your own feelings. Teasing out what you really feel and communicating it may demand a different sort of patience than you are used to. The walk provides an activity to go along with the dialogue without distracting you from the main point, giving you a sort of music or beat to measure your speech against. You'll find you can use the silence and the tap, tap, tap of your feet hitting the ground to try on different feelings and ways of expressing them before you actually say them, the way a good sales attendant can bring you different sets of clothes to try on before buying them.

Natural Communication: Listening

When we are trying to sort out issues in a relationship, we're usually so full of our own hurts and upset that we don't listen very effectively. An impatient and ill-considered retort has derailed many an attempt to repair a relationship. When you hear something that stirs up your anger, your natural response is to lash out. But when you are walking, you can take a few steps first, and breathe before responding. The natural cleansing action of the active body will take the edge off the intense feelings.

Why did a comment cause you to feel such anger? You may find that you are actually upset because you feel hurt that your partner or loved one would say such a thing. You might find after taking a few more steps that you feel hurt because you are afraid there is some truth in what she or he said but don't know how to handle seeing that in yourself. The movements of walking and breathing keep your body fluid and changing instead of rigid and closed. There are things about yourself you can hear while walking that you would find much more difficult to hear sitting in a chair, inside.

An old Irish proverb advises, "We have two ears and one mouth for a reason, so we can listen twice as much as we talk." Listening is important if you want to encourage your loved one to articulate his or her thoughts and feelings, particularly the deeper, more private ones. People are much more likely to tell you things that are hard or scary to say if they feel you being an open, attentive, and supportive listener. Love flourishes in an environment where there is emotional safety, and listening to your partner with love and care is the surest way to communicate that her or his deepest feelings and secrets are safe with you. Here are a few simple guidelines to help you listen:

- Stay objective. If your partner hesitates or feels uncomfortable communicating his or her feelings, you can repeat back what you hear or say something such as "Tell me more about that."
- Use supportive statements to maintain a positive connection. Try any of the following: "Uh-huh." "I understand." "You make sense to me."
- Don't interrupt with associative conversations ("That reminds me of a time . . .") or with advice. Your loved one needs to be heard, and premature advice can often be interpreted as a judgment or a message that what the person is feeling is not valid. Give advice only when asked for it.
- Empathize with your partner whenever possible. Let your partner know that you understand how he or she feels.

Natural Communication: Speaking

Yoga is defined as both equilibrium and skillfulness in action and, in working out a relationship, yoga is the practice of tolerating your feelings so you can respond skillfully instead of reactively. In our retreats we teach that beneath every hurt feeling is a deeper fear. Let the motion and pace of walking and breathing give you a chance to communicate your fears and insecurities as often as you do your anger and hurt.

Communicating this way lets your partner know who you are, independent of how he or she hurt or angered you. Only by knowing those sides of you can your loved one learn to be with you as you really are, without being afraid of being hurt herself or himself.

Speaking your secrets while walking lets you hear yourself with your whole being. Speaking is a function of the left brain, and hearing is a function of the right brain. When you give voice to what is hidden while walking, you give both sides of your brain and your whole being a chance to integrate the words and feelings.

As you walk, let the forward movement lend you courage in your speaking. Without courage and risk, there is no resolution or intimacy. Courageous communication contains two parts. First you must have the guts to be vulnerable, to own your fears and anxieties, and to communicate your ownership of them to the other person. For example, "I am afraid if I don't keep up with you, you will leave me. That's why I compete with you and get jealous of your successes."

Second, you must have the courage to discuss frankly the hurtful actions of your loved one. This is harder than it sounds. Even when difficult discussions seem close to being resolved, in our bellies we may still believe the other person is getting off somehow yet hesitate to express this feeling because he or she may become upset and we'll lose all the good feelings we've generated up to then. It is tempting to think, "I'm not going to make more waves, maybe this will go away over time," effectively silencing and repressing the associated feelings.

But taking the easy route robs you of true honesty in the relationship and also robs you of true resolution of the issue at hand. When you take the risk of bringing up hurtful action, you give the other person a chance to shed light on it and change your perspective. You also give the other person a chance to see some truth in your speaking and to make changes that can bring the two of you closer.

Sharing your thoughts and feelings with your loved one is critical for a long and satisfying relationship. Here are some guidelines to help you articulate what's in your mind and heart:

- Make sure there is enough time for both of you to express yourselves.
- Make "I" statements whenever possible. For example, instead of saying, "People often feel disconnected in a relationship when there isn't time for intimacy," say, "I feel disconnected from you lately because we haven't made time for each other." "I" statements are much more powerful and will help you communicate your points more effectively.
- Try to be specific and to differentiate what you observe from what you imagine, and what you feel from what you want. For example, tell the initiating event, such as, "Your mother asked if she could visit us last weekend and you said yes." Next tell the feelings that came up for you: "I felt upset with you because you had promised me a weekend without social commitments." Next tell the conclusion you drew: "You don't seem to prioritize time for us and I imagine you don't care about our relationship as much as you used to." Finally tell what you want: "I would like to save one weekend per month when we don't have company or social obligations. Is this okay with you?"
- Take your time. Go slowly enough to deliver your message with depth, clarity, and honesty.
- Consider your motivation for sharing. This process works when your intention is to gain a deeper understanding of yourself and the other person. If you are trying to make your partner wrong or make yourself look better, you won't get the personal growth benefit and you certainly won't draw your partner closer to you.

For more information about communication tools for relationships, you can read Dr. Harville Hendrix's book *Getting the Love You Want: A*

Guide for Couples or *The Secret of Staying in Love* by John Powell, which provides an excellent discussion of dialogue and intimacy. Dialogue is the key to bringing integration and unity to your relationships. In *The Miracle of Dialogue*, Reuel Howe says, "Dialogue is to love what blood is to the body. When the flow of blood stops, the body dies. When communication stops, love dies and resentment and separation are born." Making time for dialogue and connection through walking yoga is a powerful and enjoyable way to maintain healthy and intimate relationships with family members, friends, and others.

Walking for Intimacy, Connection, and Romance

If we view yoga as the practice of integrating that which is separate from us, then in many ways intimacy is both a practice and a test of yoga. A teacher of ours used to say, "You never meet anyone but yourself." If you can love one person, you can love everyone. Some spiritual seekers proclaim their love for humanity but have a great deal of trouble with people. As you practice becoming more intimate with your loved ones, you are practicing yoga. If you pay very close attention you can see that those traits you react to in others are also in you, and that in learning about the other person you are making better friends with yourself.

Walking with a friend or loved one not only gives you a chance to resolve issues between you but can also be a time to sort out your priorities, plan your future, articulate your values, rekindle romance, or just plain have fun. We personally take time on our walks to play the role of sounding board for each other, to help sort out issues that aren't necessarily between us but are in relation to work, parents, siblings, and so on. In addition, we'll periodically take time to ask these questions: "Are we doing what we want to be doing in life?" and "Is our lifestyle in line with our vision and values or are we simply being dragged along by the crush of everyday demands?"

Tips for Walking with Loved Ones

- Before you start your walk, take several minutes to warm up the body with a few Neck Rolls, Yoga Mudra, and Cobra, as described in Chapter 3, to open the chest and heart, and a Forward Bend to stretch the whole body.

- Whenever possible, plan to walk where you won't be distracted or interrupted by neighbors or traffic.

- Pick a place to walk that is surrounded by trees, grass, water, or open sky. If you live in the suburbs or the country, find the nearest state or town park. Quiet country roads with little traffic work well too. If you live in the city, try to find the nearest city park or plan to take a drive up to the country once or twice a month. You will be amazed at the natural landscapes that are within your reach. Simply get a map or call your local chamber of commerce to inquire about good places to walk near you. Your local library should have resources that list all the parks and city-run recreation areas in your vicinity.

- Walking in nature is especially conducive for couples who want to develop intimacy and rekindle romance. Try to pick locations that include an aerobic uphill climb surrounded by lots of trees and water. Taking a challenging hike brings you closer together because the physical workout makes you feel good in your body, mind, and spirit. In addition, the fresh air, the sound of running water, and the deep green of the trees have a deeply nurturing and uplifting effect on the body that is hard to get in any other circumstance. When you feel good about yourself, you automatically open up and feel closer to the person sharing your experience. Talking about more intimate issues in such a setting is much easier and more organic.

- Try to set aside at least 2 to 3 hours for the walk. It takes time to unwind and disconnect from your life and to synchronize your energy with that of your friend or loved one. In addition, if you want to have a more in-depth conversation, you need time to mine your thoughts and feelings. There are often many layers to peel off before you get to what's at the heart of the matter.

Nurturing Intimacy

At least twice a month for twelve years of our marriage we have hiked up a wonderful trail on Race Brook Mountain in the southern Berkshires of Massachusetts. The landscape of this hike, which includes steep uphill climbs, resting spots, and long, flat plateaus, perfectly facilitates the stages we need to go through to open the doors for deeper connection and communication.

The trail starts out relatively flat and skirts the northern edge of a beautiful open field leading to an entrance in the woods that feels like a portal into a world of wildness and beauty. We hold hands, take deep gulps of the fresh, scented air, and prepare ourselves mentally for the uphill climb of about seven hundred feet. We are generally silent as we climb so we can focus our attention on meeting our bodies' intense demand for oxygen and on finding a good pace.

At the top of the climb is a rock shelf where we always stop to drink some water and look out into the valley below us. The natural break in the walk functions as a transition point, where we move from the individual focus of intense physical exertion into a space in which we begin to interact with each other. The high we feel from the exercise and our surroundings gives each of us a feeling of strength and well-being from which to interact with the other.

Continuing on, we slow our pace to experience the intimacy of the moment and to let the rhythm of our walking allow what lies between us bubble up into words. One of us always has something he or she wants to talk about. Usually it is a feeling or an issue that needs time to be expressed and now feels the room and the safety to come forth. The simplicity of nature frees us to unravel the complexity of our feelings, making them seem genuine and fitting. In *The Complete Walker*, Colin Fletcher describes the experience: "It is as if my mind, set free by space and solitude and oiled by the body's easy rhythm, swings open and releases thoughts it has already formulated."

When our feelings are particularly painful or embarrassing, we take time to hesitate, test, and then slowly reveal what is in our hearts. When the walking interferes with intimacy, we take time to hang out on a rock near the stream to give space for deeper emotions to emerge.

At some point we transition from our more intimate conversation into a light and easy banter, turning our attention to the next phase of the climb. We start our final ascent with a feeling that all is well with the world. Our pace accelerates, anticipating the view from the top of the mountain and how good our lunch will taste. Walking with your beloved nurtures a sense of romance, adventure, and intimacy and will assure a long-lasting friendship.

Ila

Walking and Family Time

When you have a family, it is often difficult to find quality time together in which you can unwind, debrief, share your stories, and take time to listen to one another. By the time everybody gets home from work and school, you are too exhausted to do much more than eat, complete a few errands and chores, get homework done, and get ready for bed. Family contact time usually happens in front of the television or over a meal.

One way to connect as a family is to drive to a local park or hiking trail and take a walk or hike. Most kids don't like to walk, so you have to get creative with them. Kids do love water, rock formations, and waterfalls, and they love to get dirty exploring a challenging climb. You can walk along a beach, in a city park, or along a mountain stream, but if possible leave the beaten path and find something unusual for your kids to explore or make up games to engage them while you walk.

Ila's experience in getting her nephews from Brooklyn to walk may help you get creative with your kids. "My parents live in a fairly tame and manicured natural setting on the side of a Mountain ski resort in Vermont. I wanted to go for a walk with my nephews who were visiting, but the paved uphill roads were way too boring for them, so I had to come up with a way to entice them. Just as they started to protest about the walk, we climbed into this streambed that ran beside a condo development. Poplar trees lined the small stream, and a canopy of green leaves covered us. There were good-sized rocks for climbing over strewn through the riverbed, and we were soaked with mud and water by the time we came out at a small bridge about five hundred feet away. It wasn't a long walk, but it was very exciting.

"My four-year-old nephew, who refuses to walk anywhere, insisted that he climb up this riverbed without any help from me. Some of the rocks were bigger than he was, but he was determined to follow his older brother into the seemingly vast wilderness and explore this unusual and exciting landscape on his own. At the end of the climb, we loitered in the woods for an hour or more, enjoying each other's company and reveling in our triumph over this mighty river. I had managed to lure these wonderful little imps away from the television and other electronic gadgets by finding a walk more exciting than Pokémon."

The promise of swimming always entices kids to walk somewhere, so try to find a place to walk that has a lake, waterfall, or ocean as a reward at the end. Pretending you are explorers, American Indian trackers, or animals helps to keep younger kids interested on longer walks. For older kids, a hike that tests their skill in climbing and tones and strengthens their bodies can help to lure them away from the phone, computer, or television.

CONTEMPLATIVE WALKING

Contemplative walking is the alter ego of full-on-walking. It mirrors the focus on breath and sensation but is at the other end of the exertion scale. In contemplative walking you achieve yoga, or integration, by slowing everything down, deeply relaxing, and focusing all your awareness inward. Buddhist and Christian practitioners prescribe contemplative walking as a method for extending the time spent in meditation, and in fact it can be understood best as a form of walking meditation. When you meditate, you deeply relax your body, consciously calm your mind, and practice letting go of your usual mental processes, in which each thought chases the tail of the one before it. If you've ever practiced meditation, you will recognize a typical chain of uninterrupted thought:

"Focusing on my breath, in and out."

"I hope I can stay comfortable in this position for a while."

"Wonder what's for lunch today."

"Oops, I'm thinking, bring my attention back to the breath."

"My leg is starting to hurt."

"I wonder how much longer the meditation will last."

"These sessions seem to get longer and longer."

"I wish the teacher would end them sooner."

"My leg has fallen asleep and it really hurts, but if I move it, people will know how little I practice at home."

"When is this damn session going to end?"

When you practice contemplative walking, you might start with a similar chain of thoughts: focusing on your breath, noticing your body, miscellaneous thoughts floating through your head, but because your body is engaged and comfortable, it is easier to stay focused in the present moment. Instead of becoming preoccupied with the discomfort of the body, you are able to move into the space between your thoughts. You let the sensations of breathing and the awareness of your body rule your mind, so awareness soaks up the energy usually devoted to thinking. During walking meditation it is easier to let thoughts go and fall more deeply into relaxation.

When you practice contemplative walking, you focus on being in the present moment, enjoying each step you take. Your awareness is inward, embodying the attitude "I have nowhere to go, nothing to do, no one I have to be right now." Since you are not going anywhere in particular, every movement is slowed way down. Whereas in full-on walking you might take six to eight steps for every inhalation, in contemplative walking you might take one to three. You practice absorption in the movement and the coordination of that movement with your breath.

Absorption defines yoga, and when you absorb yourself in contemplative walking you start to create the benefits of yoga. You will find that you enter a place of peace and contentment as you walk. In addition, absorption in the present moment triggers a physiological process in which your blood pressure lowers and your muscles relax. The physiologist R. Keith Wallace and the Harvard research fellow Herbert Benson were the first to study the benefits of meditation and its effect on stress-related illness. They discovered what Dr. Benson would subsequently refer to as the relaxation response, an inducible, physiological state of quietude in which the heart rate, metabolic rate, and breathing rate drop.

Their experiments showed that during meditation the body moves into a restful state called hypometabolism, in which a marked decrease in the body's oxygen consumption occurs. Meditators were also found to experience an increased production of alpha waves or slow brain waves, which are associated with a state of relaxation, as well as a decrease in the production of blood lactate, which has been linked to anxiety. The blood pressure of meditators who had previously experienced elevated blood pressure decreased during meditation and with regular practice remained low before, during, and after the meditation sessions. When your mind is focused through meditation or walking yoga, you can counteract the effects of stress and connect with the body's own powerful ability to heal and rejuvenate itself. Contemplative walking is an effective practice to tap into your own relaxation response, especially if you don't have the temperament to meditate sitting still.

Contemplative walking can be used for many reasons. On a practical level contemplative walking is very helpful when you get so agitated that you can't face sitting and meditating, and you need some sort of movement in which to absorb yourself. Some of our students use just five minutes of their lunch break to practice contemplative walking so they can completely disconnect from the hustle and bustle of the office. Many people have reported to us that they overcome creative blocks just by taking a fifteen-minute break for slow contemplative walking, during which they can rest from thinking. Perhaps most beneficial is the relaxing and calming effect of contemplative walking on the body.

For thousands of years spiritual seekers have used walking as a metaphor for connecting to the sacred or as a tool for developing insight and mastery of the mind. Zen Buddhists intersperse periods of sitting meditation with *kinhin*, or walking meditation. Jesuit monks repeat the rosary during meditation walks in the ambulatories of their monasteries. The labyrinth, which exists in many cultures, has been used in the Christian tradition as a symbolic journey or as a map a seeker can actually follow, symbolizing a move from the outer, worldly life to the inner, sacred life. The common denominator that flows through the many variations of contemplative walking is the desire to find some form of personal enlightenment or inner peace and a sense of integration with the world around us.

Whether you use contemplative walking to bring a deeper spiritual dimension to your life or as a tool for stress management, the methods are simple. The primary goal of meditation is to experience synchronicity of body and mind, so you are completely present with whatever is going on in the moment. Through regular practice you develop the capacity to observe your thoughts, emotions, and physical sensations objectively, without judgment or reaction. The practice of meditation helps us go through life's ups and downs, hopes and fears, with courage, strength, and contentment. Contemplative walking is one way to learn to meditate without the physical discomfort of sitting meditation.

Keeping the mind focused in the present moment is much harder than it sounds. You will find that, within a few seconds of attempting to concentrate on the breath or physical sensations, a thought will carry you away completely. Before you know it, you are dreaming of your summer vacation instead of being aware of placing one foot in front of the other.

One technique you can use to help disengage from thinking is to see your thoughts as helium balloons on strings. As soon as you become aware of holding a string, let it go, and allow the thought to float away like a balloon. Sometimes you can use an image or set of words to go back to when your thoughts carry you away. Mantras (see page 135) are simple phrases that help let thoughts drift away. Labeling your thoughts as "thinking" gives you tremendous leverage in bringing your awareness back to your breath. In other words, when you find yourself absorbed in a thought, simply repeat the word *thinking* to yourself as a way to objectify the thought and withdraw its power over you. As you practice you will discover you get better at seeing your thoughts form and then float away, and when this happens you start to gain a new perspective on life. You watch your thoughts form and disperse and you realize that *you* are watching, and *you* are separate from your thoughts! What does it mean to realize *you* are separate from your thoughts?

When Heather first came to one of our walking yoga retreats, she felt beset by stress and worry. Heather had two children, and she constantly imagined all manner of dire disasters befalling them. This concern bred even more stress because her children rebelled against her incessant worry and had begun to act out in ways that caused Heather even more strain. As Heather started to practice contemplative walking, she got some distance between herself and her worry. She saw that she spent almost all her energy being anxious about things that never happened. Heather watched her mind manufacture future catastrophes one after another without pause, regardless of the likelihood of them ever happening. Once she was familiar with her pattern, she could start to practice releasing those thoughts instead of obsessing over them.

Heather still worries about her children, but she can see through the worry and reach a place of connection with herself beyond the learned pattern of anxiety. Now when Heather starts worrying, she can say, "Oh, I'm in my worry pattern again, let me take a few deep breaths and relax. Let me go back to that place I go to when I do my contemplative walking, where I can see my worry objectively so that it loses its control over me."

Practicing Contemplative Walking

You can practice contemplative walking in any size space, inside or outside, alone or with a group. Try to follow a path or a set route so you don't have to put your energy into navigation. Inside your house pick a room for practice, preferably with the least amount of furniture, and walk a set path, a circle or a square. You can also practice outdoors, following a walking path in your backyard or in a park.

Before you start your contemplative walking yoga, take a few minutes to warm up your body with a routine that might include Neck Rolls, Butterfly pose, Knee to Chest pose, Knee Down Twist, and Child pose, as described in Chapter 3.

- Stand for a moment at the beginning of the path you plan to follow.
- Bring your body into Mountain pose (see page 59).
- Gaze softly in front of you, with your hands at your sides.
- Start to take long, deep breaths using Ujjayi breath (see page 101).
- Begin the crosslateral movement: As you inhale take a step forward with your right foot, planting your heel on the ground and rolling onto your toes, swinging your left arm at the same time. As you exhale, swing your left leg and right arm forward and continue to alternate your steps and arm swings in coordination with your breath. You can moderate your pace to be as slow as one step per breath or as fast as three steps per breath.
- Focus the mind by counting breaths and paying attention to the sensations of your body. Whenever you find yourself absorbed in the stories of your thoughts, let them go by imagining that your thoughts are balloons filled with helium.
- Be sure to stay relaxed during this exercise. Relax your face, your shoulders, your abdomen, and your hands. Remember you have

nowhere to go, nothing to do, and no one to be. Allow your breath to help you sink into the experience of living in the present moment.

We recommend practicing for at least 10 to 15 minutes at a time, especially if you are using contemplative walking as an alternative to sitting meditation.

WALKING WITH GRATITUDE

Full-on-walking and contemplative walking both deal with finding yoga—union—by focusing your awareness on the breath and sensations of your body, though each does so in a different way. Another way of finding that sense of connection is by extending your senses outward instead of inward, to see, smell, hear, taste, and feel the world around you with a sense of reverence, gratitude, and awe.

Native American wisdom and traditions are based on an appreciation for the natural world and our place within the circle of life. A Lakota elder once said, "Every step you take on earth should be a prayer." When you walk with gratitude, you consciously practice appreciation for being alive and surrounded by creation. You'll find that gratitude is an easy doorway to calming the restlessness of the mind. When you are grateful, you open to the possibility of being completely content with your life. You learn to approach each moment with the eyes of a child, receptive to the wonder of what life has to offer.

We had a vivid experience of how precious each moment is during a plane ride several years ago. We were coming back home from a business trip, circling the Cleveland airport to land. The day was bright and sunny, and we sat together looking forward to landing and getting this leg of the trip behind us. We still had to board another plane for the final flight to the Albany airport, from which we would drive home. We circled as planes usually do and kept losing altitude in the normal way. Everything seemed familiar. We looked down and saw the ground coming closer—it seemed to us that we were only about a thousand feet up.

Suddenly, everything changed. The plane dropped like a stone, and we were pressed against our seat belts while our stomachs seemed to rise into our throats. We looked at each other and grabbed each other's hand thinking, "This could be it." We weren't sure the plane had enough altitude to adjust to the sickening drop that had just happened. Then the plane dropped again! We've been scared before, but this was different. In a moment we added up the two drops with the nearness of the ground, and we both felt the seriousness of the scene in our cells. It sounds trite, but our lives really did flash before our eyes.

In an instant, a deep sense of love and gratitude flooded our hearts as images of our life together passed through our minds. Faces of our family flashed before us. To our surprise, we also experienced a sense of sadness. It hit us how much energy we had spent worrying about the future instead of appreciating the present. All our worries seemed so unimportant to us in that moment, and we wished we hadn't wasted so much time focused on them.

Of course, you wouldn't be reading this right now if the plane had not righted itself and landed safely, but the experience has stayed with us ever since and changed us in a profound way. For one thing, it gave us an incredible appreciation for how short life really is. When the moment came that we were possibly facing our deaths, it seemed the thirty-eight years we had lived had passed by in a few minutes. Now, for the most part, we live our lives conscious of the fact that our time here on earth is going to be over much more quickly than we can imagine, and we maintain a sense of gratitude and appreciation for all that we have.

Practicing Contentment

The practice of walking with gratitude brings more appreciation and contentment into one's life. In yoga there is a moral observance called *santosha*, contentment. This practice can be understood as the ability to tolerate the mental and physical disturbances and fluctuations that interfere with our ability to enjoy things as they are. Most of our mental and physical disturbances come from trying to get more: more money, more material things, more security, and more love. Striving for more in life is not the problem, it is the inability to be content with what we have.

John, a friend of ours, tells a great story about contentment. John didn't enjoy his work very much, so he would suffer through his morning looking forward to his daily walk at lunchtime. He loved the hour and a half that he would spend breathing in the fresh air, enjoying the lush green scenery, and getting a good workout. All year he would dream about his summer vacation, when he could live outdoors and take relaxing walks for as many hours as he pleased, with no work to interfere with his relaxation.

Finally his vacation came, and he packed up his family and took off for a two-week vacation to the White Mountains of New Hampshire. The first day was the most enjoyable day he had experienced in a long time. He was thrilled not to have to go to work, and he and his family took a long hike after a delicious breakfast that tasted so much better because they were eating it in the great outdoors. It took several hours to hike to the top of the mountain, with the family frequently stopping to pick wild blueberries, examine local plant life, and look for signs of wildlife. For John, though, the peak experience of the day came at the top of the mountain, where he enjoyed hundred-mile vistas in every direction.

John was so taken with this experience that the next day he rushed the family through breakfast so they could get an earlier start. It still took several hours to get to the top of the mountain because they spent time resting and snacking along the steep uphill climb, but eventually they came to the peak, where he could enjoy the great long-distance views.

Each day John felt more and more impatient with the preparations of the camp, making of the meals, and even the hiking they had to do to get to the top of the mountain. He rushed his family through their breakfasts and then pushed everyone so that the hiking became more of a forced march. He began to dislike every part of the hike except the part when he could sit at the top of the mountain and enjoy the views.

At the end of the first week, his wife began to cry and pointed out to him how he was ruining their vacation in the name of getting to sit at the top of the mountain. Suddenly, it hit him: He was re-creating the experience of his day-to-day life on his vacation. He had set himself up to enjoy only about an hour and a half of his day. It wasn't preparing breakfast, hiking, or work that was the problem, it was his inability to find contentment in each moment.

The yogis say that the habits of the mind bring great suffering but that the mind has one primary advantage: It will always return to what is familiar to it. When you habituate your mind to be appreciative and grateful, your whole life takes on a greater degree of sustaining spirituality. There are many ways to cultivate a sense of gratitude to take with you on your walks: sitting for a moment in appreciation of the abundance on your table before eating, beginning or ending your day with a small prayer of thanks, or expressing appreciation to a friend or colleague are just a few.

John Lennon once said, "Life is what happens to you while you are busy making other plans." It is important, in the midst of all our planning and striving, to make some time to enjoy what we have. Walking with gratitude can help develop contentment by training the mind to be satisfied with simple pleasures. This kind of walking is also helpful when you are going through a crisis of faith or a period of anxiety. When you feel alone and alienated from the world and other people, go for a walk with the intention of opening to the sensation of gratitude and allow your faith to be renewed. Whether you are walking on the bustling streets of Manhattan or on an empty country lane, there is always something to appreciate. Every step can bring you a new experience.

The Web of Life

Albert Einstein has been quoted as saying, "The highest point a man can attain is not knowledge, or virtue, or goodness, or victory, but something even greater and more heroic: Sacred Awe!" At a fundamental level, human life exists as part of an ecosystem of exchange of oxygen and carbon dioxide, our lives literally feeding plant life and they in return feeding us. Each and every species of life exists within a miraculous web of interconnected relationships.

Recently on one of our daily walks, we saw a dead fawn on the side of the road. It was heartbreaking to see the tender young deer mangled by the impact of a car, its life snuffed out so quickly. But life and death are perfect partners. Over the next few days we watched as nature's recycling process took place. First the crows ate the meat of the body, then the flies came, then the maggots, devouring every bit of nutrition. Within five days all the flesh of deer had been used to sustain some form of life. The bones, skin, and hair remained drying in the sun, eventually to be reabsorbed into the earth and used as nourishment for the plant life along the road.

When you walk with gratitude, you can sense the ever-changing and eternal dance of spirit. Everything grows and decays, and the wheels of life continuously spin. Every moment new life springs forth while old life withers and dies. When you practice walking with gratitude, you will start to see how everything is connected and that you are part of this wonderful intelligent universe.

So take a walk in which your sole purpose is be present to the amazing world we live in and let yourself walk at the nexus of life, like a thread in the infinite tapestry of being. When you walk in this way, you'll soon find it's hard to hold on to the worries and struggles that can overpower your joy in life. When life reaches out to you, you can grasp its hand and be lifted into the whole.

Practicing Walking with Gratitude

Before you start your walk, take 10 to 15 minutes to stretch your body, and include one Sun Salutation, Warrior pose, Locust, Yoga Mudra, and the Forward Bend, as described in Chapter 3. Then take 5 minutes to practice the complete yogic breath and Ujjayi breathing, as described in Chapter 4.

- Stand at the beginning of the path or road you plan to walk and notice how your feet are connected to the earth, your body standing straight and tall, perfectly balanced and connecting to the sky. Spend a moment really taking in the view around you. Like a camera, your eyes transmit images to your brain and allow you to experience the colors, shapes, distances, textures, and dimensions of the natural world. For those with the ability to see, approximately four-fifths of everything we know reaches the brain through sight. Consider the miracle of sight, and take a moment to be grateful for your ability to see.
- Focus on your ears and the sound waves in the air around you. Tune in to the sounds you hear: birds, insects, dogs, traffic, people talking, lawn mowers, and airplanes. Notice tone, volume, and rhythm as the sound waves transform into electrical signals that your brain

can "hear." In addition to carrying sound waves, your ear contains an organ that helps you balance. Take a moment to appreciate what a wonder of nature your ears are and how good it is to be able to hear and balance.

- Take a deep breath in though your nose and notice the smells around you. Some smells make your mouth water, some intoxicate, some repulse. Taste the air around you, and appreciate the sensations of taste and smell.

- Last, close your eyes and notice the sensation of the air around you tickling the hairs on your skin. Your skin is the largest organ of your body and provides you with a very sophisticated layer of protection. Feel the pleasure of the wind on your face and take a minute to appreciate your skin, that amazing transporter of sensation.

- Begin your walk using the crosslateral motion. Swing your right leg forward, stepping onto your heel; roll forward onto the ball of the right foot; balance on the ball and toes of the right foot, and push off with the big toe of the left foot as you swing your left leg forward. Your right arm swings forward at the same time as your left leg, as if an internal hinge connects them. Breathe deeply using Ujjayi breathing and start noticing as many sensations as possible. When you take a walk with gratitude, be sure to look up and around, not down at your feet. It is so easy to get lost in thought and not even notice where you are or what you are doing. Paying attention to your surroundings and attuning all your senses to your experience will make each moment rich with pleasure.

Imagine yourself as an ancient one in the tradition of the American Indian; make each step a prayer, and walk in gratitude for the earth and your life. Allow your sense of time to expand and blend in with the timeless rhythms of the earth, thinking in terms of millennia instead of hours.

Chapter 6

walking to places of peace and power

Where you walk is important. There is an elemental connection you feel when you walk next to a river, hill, or glen that you don't get when the environment has been paved over. For millions of years humans have walked to places where nature's voice is dominant. We are first and foremost creatures birthed in the womb of the planet we live on. We are products of nature, inextricably tied to the earth. Our genes have nature coded within them, and our cells remember. Whether we walk by a deep river, an ocean shoreline, a splashing secret glen, an ancient mountain, or a special grove of trees, something in our cellular memory awakens in places of natural power. We experience something elemental and larger than ourselves, and in some unspoken way our souls respond to that deep-toned rumble of nature's voice. We feel soothed and renewed. We come home to ourselves.

John Muir, the great naturalist responsible for helping to get our national park system in place, probably said it best when he wrote, "Go into the mountains and receive their good tidings." He phrased it this way because he knew the experience to be active on both parts. We need to "go into the mountains"—to surround ourselves with nature. Notice that he said "go into," not just "go to." We are not looking *at* but *being in*. "Receive their good tidings"—nature will speak if we will listen.

However, listening to and understanding nature's intelligence requires us first to slow down to attune to nature's rhythms.

Consciously walking in nature is yoga. Whenever we practice listening to the greater intelligence of the universe we are practicing yoga, whether we listen inside to the pulse of breath and blood or we listen outside to the workings of life expressed in the song of the bird and the splash of the waterfall. Yoga's aim is to experience ourselves as we truly are, without the constant mental chatter of hankering and fear, past and future. Any practice that silences this chatter is yoga. Surrounded by nature, our minds leap beyond the purely personal, separated world and tap into a larger, more integrated world.

Walking is an integral part of the practice, because you can't join in union with nature any other way. Many people tour national parks by car, but their experience of powerful places can be compared more to watching a video. There is no real connection to nature when it is viewed from a moving vehicle. Steel and plastic somehow interfere with the rhythms of stone and stream. Even a bicycle clatters around a bit between you and the dance of soil, sun, air, and water. When you walk, you place yourself *there*. You go *into* the mountains. Why is this such a distinct experience?

We are most human when we are walking. Walking upright differentiates us from all other species on the planet and is a trait that most humans share. Walking connects us to one another and to our ancestors. For most of human history, we have wandered on foot. Whether out of necessity or curiosity, humans have traveled, following the seasonal flight of birds and the movements of migratory herds, or simply following an inner urge to explore.

When you walk you are in your natural body, moving across the earth, embodying the animal part of yourself embedded in you over millennia. All the evolution contained in your cellular memory comes alive when you walk in nature. Echoes of the entire experience of life on the planet come alive with each step you take away from the settled village and into the wild lands.

Indigenous people all over the world understand the power of our relationship to the natural world. When we spend time in nature, particularly in the wild, untamed parts of nature, we experience a connection to something much bigger than ourselves, something so intelligent and magnificent in its being that it gives us a glimpse of our own true nature. Something very primal and sacred happens in nature. It has the power to silence the mind and fill us with awe.

Many ancient cultures had rituals and rites of passage in which members ventured into nature to learn about themselves. They tied the great transitions of life to rituals that tapped into the wisdom of the great mother earth. For instance, American Indians sent their adolescent boys out on vision quests. The adolescent would leave the village as a boy, live alone in the wilderness for several days, and return as a man only after the vision for his life had appeared. Native people know that when you walk into nature you mute the discord in your own mind and amplify the intelligence available in creation. What happens when you do this? Your body, mind, and spirit begin to return to their natural state. Stress, resistance, fear, and worry diminish as your rhythms slow down and tune in to nature's flow.

All things in nature are sympathetic. All parts of nature exist in a distinct vibratory field, and when those fields contact one another, their vibrations tend to match. For example, women who live close together begin to menstruate at the same time each month, and when you listen to music with a catchy beat, your foot starts to tap and your body naturally moves with the pulse.

Exactly the same thing happens when you walk into nature. From a yogic perspective, the entire universe is intelligent, and that intelligence is working both inside us and in the natural world. In yoga, to truly know oneself is to know oneself as part of the boundless web of intelligent existence. Yogis often describe the relationship of the individual soul to the vast universe by using the metaphor of individual waves in a vast ocean. Each of the waves seems to be separate, but in reality they are all part of the same ocean. As in the microcosm, so in the macrocosm. Each of us has at our core the same resonant melody that pervades all of nature. When you walk to places of natural power, you surround yourself with the music that plays most naturally in your soul. Your inner being responds by damping the discord of fear, worry, and separation and starts falling into harmony with its core vibrations.

All music and rhythm derive their meaning and beauty from the interweaving of sound and silence and the interrelationship of high and low notes. We could say our lives gain their meaning and beauty in the same way. Each one of us goes through ups and downs, periods of expression and periods of withdrawal, experiences of joy and wonder changing to experiences of loss and hurt. Through these patterns our lives are wrought and our wisdom gained.

In nature there are seasons, and to each season there is a purpose. When you visit a grove of trees in the fall and marvel at their fiery foliage, you never get the feeling that the trees are standing around worrying about the coming winter and mourning the loss of their leaves. Imagine the absurdity of two of the trees off in a corner discussing the tragedy of Mary the Maple, who died in last year's frost. The vibration of the forest is not like that at all. When we are in the presence of a forest of trees, the ebb and flow of life seems so fitting and natural, the long winter hibernation simply the final act following the brilliant crescendo in the yearly cycle.

If our core melody is harmonious and integrative, why do we ever fall into discord and separation? Unfortunately, we often lose that sense of acceptance and celebration in all our seasons of life. We fall into the place where we crave certain types of experiences and fear others. We have a joyful time and want to have more and more of those kinds of feelings. We have a hard time and set about making sure we'll never have another if we can help it. We start to steer our lives by greed for more fun and fear of more pain, and in so doing become separated from our natural pace. When we steer our lives by these twin variables of attraction and aversion, we set ourselves in opposition to the natural rhythms of nature and thus fall out of tune with the larger song going on around us.

When we walk to places where nature predominates, we give ourselves a chance to remember who we really are. In nature there is nowhere to go and nothing to do. Greed and fear have little hold on our minds because there is no goal or dissatisfaction in the being of an ocean or a mountain. They merely are as they are, basking in the limitless now. When you go to them, they will share their peace if you ask.

Every year we spend time in the wilderness of the Sierra Nevada as a way to unplug, recharge, and gain perspective on life. It has become a pilgrimage of sorts, in which our walk into the mountains acts as a metaphor for a journey into the sacred. For us time in the wilderness, during which we can witness life from its inception and see a history that is hundreds of thousands of years old, has a transformative power that is as real as that of any religion. When you stand deep in the heart of the Sierras, thousands of feet above sea level, you get an incredibly big view, both physically and psychologically. The experience leaves no doubt that there is something much greater than humankind at work and imparts a sense that you can trust your life to a larger wisdom. We actively use our time in the mountains to shape the long view of our lives, set new directions, celebrate major life passages and accomplishments, let go of our past, and renew lifelong vows.

In his book *Walden*, Henry David Thoreau talks about why he chose to spend time in the wilderness: "I went to the woods because I wished to live deliberately, to front only the essential facts of life, and see if I could not learn what it had to teach, and not, when I came to die, discover that I had not lived." Spending time in nature and contemplating life's deeper meaning is not just for philosophers; you too can follow the call of the wild simply by walking into places of peace and power.

Time and Nature

Can our problems exist outside of time? We've all suffered through tough and painful experiences: deaths, divorces, and breakdowns. A large part of the suffering we experience comes from that terrible feeling that life is going to stay like that forever. Connecting with the eternal flow of nature's time helps us to put things into perspective. Our problems may still exist, and probably do, but we have changed in relation to them.

When Frank came to our workshop, he had just lost his job because the company he worked for decided to downsize. Frank had worked there for fifteen years and thought he might work there for many more. Losing his job was devastating to him. He wasn't sure what he would do next and came to our walking yoga workshop as a way to gain some perspective. What was most difficult for Frank was his fear of the future and the unknown. He shared that he was haunted by thoughts of never working again, and never being valuable to a business. What if he couldn't find a new job? What if his feelings of inadequacy deepened and remained with him, undermining his confidence and thereby affecting his interviewing skills?

We suggested that Frank spend some time in nature near flowing water, letting the eternal quality of the stream soak into him. The Buddhists find wisdom in meditating on the impermanence of all things, contemplating the thought that all things must change. We knew nature would provide some of that sense for Frank. We wanted him to have a chance to see his challenges against a larger span of time, in this case the stream's long history, to get a sense of himself beyond his most recent setback.

Unlike us, nature is neither striving nor resisting, nor does it have deadlines to meet and futures to gain or avoid. One of the most salient vibrations you can feel when walking in wild places is the sense of timelessness. There is no rush, no squeezing of tasks into a finite amount of time. The ocean has always been there, so too the mountains. When you go into such places, it's hard to let the problems of the day dominate your mind. Nature is moving in too grand a cycle for that. When you see your daily struggles against the movement of aeons in nature, you automatically diminish their power over you. The comparison always shrinks your self-discouraging worries.

If you can taste nature's timelessness on a regular basis, you will find that it starts to be a part of your perspective on life. You begin to embody that same rhythm and pace all the time, and your life starts to gain a sense of ease and relaxation. Whether it is the top of a mountain, the base of a waterfall, the edge of a large field, or the roots of a favorite tree, when you walk to places of peace and power, stop and take in their magic. The more you return to a place of peace and power, the more you imbue it with your own vibrations, and it begins to speak to you more clearly.

Ceremonies in Nature

There is something very magical about places of peace and power; they lend themselves to ceremonies, rites, rituals, and celebrations of all kinds. A ceremony or ritual is a simple way to formalize commitments, honor transitions, or celebrate accomplishments. These acts uplift our spirits, give us a way to acknowledge the ones we love, and help us call upon forces greater than ourselves to witness and bless our endeavors. Baptisms, bat mitzvahs, funerals, and weddings are ceremonies based on social traditions. We can also introduce more personal rituals and ceremonies into our everyday lives. They need not be elaborate to be effective; use your inner knowing and imagination to create moments of magic.

Places of peace and power in nature offer ideal settings for performing a small ceremony or ritual. We perform several rituals during our annual backpacking trip into the wilderness of the Sierra Mountains in Northern California. With these simple rites we fulfill different purposes, such as a renewal of our marriage vows, prayers to receive the blessings of the great mother, and setting our intentions for the coming year.

We perform one such ritual just over Catherine Lake pass, which is at about 13,000 feet above sea level and forms the entryway to a small circular sanctuary at the base of Mounts Ritter and Banner. It takes about four days of steady hiking to get to this isolated location, which seems a perfect place to perform a ritual because of its breathtaking beauty and absolute silence. The glacier-fed lake just below the pass is filled with pure, sparkling blue-green water, the perfect ingredient for our ceremony. The ritual is a simple one in which we use water to bless each other and purify our bodies.

First each of us cups some water in our hands and sprinkles it on the other's head reciting the words "In the presence of the earth mother, the mountain gods, the wind, and sky, may this water purify and strengthen you." Next we each cup some water in our hands and drink it, reciting the words "May the water of life nourish you and keep you safe from harm."

A Ceremony in Nature

Many years ago we ran across a party of four seasoned hikers deep in the heart of the Ansel Adams Wilderness near Yosemite National Park carrying what looked like a very small casket. You usually don't see people with anything but backpacks, so we asked them what they were doing. The container held the ashes of their good friend and hiking companion who had died several months earlier. The son and friends of this man were carrying the old hiker to his final resting place high in the Sierras. They planned to perform an informal ceremony to express their love and bid farewell to their beloved comrade and leave him where he could be free to roam the hills and streams.

HOW TO DESIGN YOUR OWN CEREMONY

You can create the content of your ceremony as you walk, letting its design come to you from the trees, the wind, and the earth. Collect natural items you find along your way, such as water, leaves, feathers, stones, flowers, and fruit; you may also want to bring along matches and a candle or some incense.

When you arrive at your formal spot, find a place to sit comfortably and spend a few minutes arranging your ceremonial materials in front of you. Then close your eyes and relax yourself by taking a few minutes to meditate, taking complete yogic breaths and using Ujjayi breathing to facilitate quieting your mind.

When you open your eyes, give yourself a moment to absorb the splendor of your surroundings. Look around you, listen to the sounds of nature, breathe in the scented air, and feel the sensation of the wind on your skin.

Next, silently or out loud, invoke the presence of the natural intelligence around you. Call on the wind, the sky, the sun, the moon and stars, the mountains, rivers, oceans, and earth. Invite the animal spirits, your ancestors, and the presence of your loved ones. Finally, call on your sacred connection to spirit.

At this point, you can perform your ceremony or ritual as you were guided to design it on your walk. Here is a simple option you may wish to build upon:

Place the flower petals, leaves, fruit, stones, and feathers in a circle in front of you to symbolize your connection to the physical world. Take time to make an arrangement of your items that is pleasing to your eyes.

Next, sprinkle water around the place you are sitting and on everyone, including yourself, to purify the ground and yourselves.

Light your candle or incense and slowly wave it in a clockwise circle to invoke knowledge, wisdom, and insight, and to create a bridge between the spiritual and the earthly worlds.

Next, do what you came to do: say your prayer, make your vows, affirm your gratitude, or honor your loved ones. Express yourself from your heart. Take your time and enjoy the moment.

When you are finished, sit quietly and meditate for a few moments to take in the sense of the sacred and allow the significance of the ceremony you have just performed to change you inside. You can step back into ordinary reality with a smile on your lips and enjoy the rest of the day.

Ceremony helps us to live our lives as we intended them and to celebrate all the different phases of life. We both believe that when you set an intention and call on the forces of nature and the universe to support you, something shifts inside, and more often than not your dreams and commitments come true.

Thoreau said, "If one advances confidently in the direction of his dreams, and endeavors to live the life which he has imagined, he will meet with a success unexpected in common hours. He will put some things behind, will pass an invisible boundary; new, universal, and more liberal laws will begin to establish themselves around and within him; or the old laws be expanded, and interpreted in his favor in a more liberal sense, and he will live with the license of a higher order of beings." Ceremony and ritual help us advance confidently in the direction of our dreams, and performing them in places of peace and power lend them a sense of promise and good fortune.

Chapter 7

yoga and walking for life

We all experience it. We promise to do something good for ourselves but when the time comes to follow through with our commitment, we don't do it. Keeping our commitment to practice often falls by the wayside because life gets in the way.

In our case, we each chose to move into an ashram at an early age because we wanted the support to follow through with our commitment to yogic lifestyle. The structured days and the like-minded community were very helpful for making the consistent practice of yoga part of our lives. For many years this worked well, we were up at 4:00 A.M. and had completed several hours of yoga, meditation, and walking before breakfast and work. But then, as the ashram grew and we took on more responsibility, worked harder, and had to deal with the real-life stresses of running the business of a large yoga center, getting up at 4:00 A.M. wasn't so easy anymore. For a while we would get up because we felt we should—there was a strong community ethic that you weren't "spiritual" if you didn't get up and do your practice—but then even that motivation failed. Our practice had become a should that our teacher had set forth in our morning scripture reading class, a competition to keep up with some community ideal, or a lofty goal, which even he didn't practice.

The changing point in our relationship to practice and self-care came when we finally stopped trying to keep up with other people or our ideals and adjusted our practice to reflect our personal circumstances. We started "sleeping in," in ashram lingo, and taking long walks at lunch break or in the evening. Each day we would follow our instincts and do what we were drawn to do. At that point, the two of us were in charge of opening a new yoga center in a 164,000-square-foot building that had been lying dormant for ten years and had to be up and running in six months. It was like resurrecting the *Titanic*. We were working long hours and dealing with more pressure and stress than we had ever handled in our lives, so naturally our practice needed to change to suit our circumstance. We needed more sleep, and we craved walking outside in the fresh air. We made walking yoga our primary practice and hatha yoga secondary, and since we needed more sleep, we shifted our practice time to our lunch or dinner break. We both realized that taking care of our health and spirit wasn't about establishing rigid practice goals that were often unrealistic and set us up to fail. Practice was about doing something we loved, something that truly nurtured us and that we could tailor to our specific lifestyle needs.

The Pleasure of Practice

I used to be a long-distance runner, and for many years I craved the feeling I would get from running. I was up at 4:00 A.M. and out on the road by 4:30 running like a deer through the quiet country roads around where I lived. I loved the feel of the wind on my face, the scent of early morning dew, and the details of the world waking up from its slumber. The regularity with which I ran came from the sheer pleasure I experienced from the exercise. The more I ran, the more I wanted to run. I would go to bed early so that I could wake up on time. I made sure that I didn't eat too much at night so I wouldn't feel sluggish in the morning. It wasn't a matter of disciplining myself; my commitment came from enjoying my experience. As I aged, my running turned to walking because that felt better for my knees and hips and was more complementary for my yoga practice. To this day my walking yoga practice is my touchstone for coming home to myself and creating a strong connection to my inner center, which nurtures and sustains me in the good times and bad.

Ila

Over time our natural urges toward health and well-being can get covered with crusty layers of bad habits, addictive behavior, and stress. When we listen to our bodies after a stressful day, they say: Pizza, television, chocolate, sugar, coffee, cigarette, wine, drugs, sleep! The messages are very basic and the cravings very strong. We have every right to feel this way. When we get home from our jobs, the work doesn't stop. The kids need us, or our spouses, or our parents, plus the laundry, grocery shopping, bills, and meal preparation all have to be tended to. Something important always calls to us, and we need a quick fix either to give us energy or to relax us. During a good week we'll squeeze in one yoga class, the occasional walk or run, or a trip to the gym.

But as we all know, the quick fix doesn't make us feel good in the long run, and the occasional workout does little to supply the energy we need to deal with the demands and stresses of life. In this chapter we will cover tips for beginning and, more important, sustaining a walking yoga practice, as well as the advantages of walking at different times of the day and different times of the year.

Getting Started with Walking Yoga

The hardest step is the first step out the door, and the best step is the last one. Even though you may be tired at the end of your walk, you feel a sense of accomplishment, your endorphins are flowing, and you have more energy for the rest of the day. If you're an evening walker, you'll feel more relaxed having washed your body of toxic stress hormones, you'll digest your dinner better, and you'll sleep more soundly. The key to getting out every day is to remember how good you will feel at the end of your walk.

COMPANY IS STRONGER THAN WILLPOWER

Group support helps keep up a practice. Find a local walking group, or partner with a friend. Our student Catherine has a standing commitment to meet someone just about every day because, as she points out, "You won't let a friend down but it is very easy to let yourself down." When you haven't made a commitment, it is simple to find excuses such as "It's too cold." "It's dark." "It's raining." "I'm too tired." However, when your focus is on the commitment to your friend, not on the exercise, you are more likely to do the exercise and get the added benefit of the camaraderie that comes with exercising together.

Participating in a retreat is also helpful to kick-start a regular walking yoga practice. When you take time out of your daily life to immerse yourself in the study and practice of yoga and walking, you can interrupt your normal habits and ways of relating to your body and mind to form a new lifestyle routine. Many runners and athletes test themselves in local and national races because the power of the group inspires their strengths to go beyond their personal limits. In the same way, when you practice yoga and walking in a group, you will often challenge yourself in ways you wouldn't by yourself. You develop a whole new level of strength and flexibility by spending several hours a day for two to five days studying and practicing. Concentrated study and practice is especially important if you are a beginner or if you haven't practiced yoga or walking in a long time. Your chances of keeping up a regular exercise routine are much greater if you deeply understand what you are doing and have uninterrupted time to practice.

For example, we have tried to learn both downhill and cross country skiing. With downhill skiing, we spent four consecutive days taking lessons from an expert and practicing. On the first day we learned to snowplow, and on the third we learned to parallel ski. By the time we left the slopes, we understood the basic principles of skiing, where to distribute our weight, how to "edge" as we skied downhill, and how to control downhill velocity. Because we had immersed ourselves in the physical and mental experience of skiing over an extended period of time, our skill had improved to a point where we were able to enjoy downhill skiing on our own and even improve our technique over time. Conversely, with cross-country skiing, we never took a lesson and would go out on our own for an hour every so often and struggle with the cross-country ski technique. To this day we can't cross-country ski. In fact, we started to hate the experience because it was so frustrating—on the uphills our skis would slide backward, and on the downhills we had absolutely no control. There were times when we would fall over standing still on a flat plain! Needless to say, our cross-country skis have been donated to a local church. Had we taken the time to learn about cross-country skiing from an experienced skier and spent some concentrated periods practicing, we are sure we would be adept by now.

Transforming Through Concentrated Practice

While I had been an occasional gym rat and had taken a few yoga classes, entering film school in my forties dismantled all my attempts at exercise or a healthy lifestyle. On the eve of my walking yoga retreat, even with a strong Buddhist practice, I was overweight, exhausted and pissed off. I also didn't think this retreat would really be any different from any other yoga class I had suffered through.

However, from the first night to the last afternoon, a very quiet and life-transforming revolution took hold. For one thing, Ila and Garrett Sarley were human beings. They understood that changing one's lifestyle was competing against grueling schedules and decades-old habits and that once we went back to the city there would be smoking and drinking and french fries. But because of this deep acceptance of whatever "real" lives we were all attached to, they opened up doors of possibilities for all of us. Ever so slowly over two days, they seduced the class into hours of yoga without anyone noticing.

By mid-morning of Saturday, my body started feeling rested, relaxed, quiet, and centered, all states I hadn't experienced much in twenty years, at least not without drugs. My knees, wrists, and back, perpetually unhappy, felt more fluid and mobile. I began to feel more energy that weekend than I had in a year of film school. By the end of the weekend, I was having epiphanies about the choices I was making in my life and how I could change.

I went back to the city and my grueling schedule brimming

with healthy plans. In fact, for about a month I stopped drinking coffee and started doing a little bit of yoga each day. And then school, work, family, holidays, and my own old habits crashed in, and walking yoga was just a pleasant weekend that had happened in the fall.

Yet I felt haunted by the Sarleys' workshop, more and more aware of how sick I was making myself by not attending to my health. After the New Year I started the slow process back. I changed my diet completely, cut back to one to two cups of coffee *a week*, started doing a little bit of yoga and walking almost every day, began to eat green vegetables, and made efforts to be more honest and straightforward. A peace and lightness began to fill my days and enhance my daily spiritual practice.

My body feels better than it has in years, and my spirit feels stronger. I'm beginning to feel physically what I have always felt inside—very much alive, peppy as all hell, and in a damn good mood.

C. O. Moed
Writer, New York City

Times of Day for Practice

EARLY MORNING

They say that people who walk in the morning are more likely to keep their commitments, because early morning, especially for parents, is the only time of day you are sure to have a free schedule. There are no doctor appointments, dance rehearsals, or softball practices to take the kids to, and no grocery shopping or other errands to keep you from your commitment to walk. Early morning is especially nice for city walkers because you have the streets to yourselves. When you walk in the morning you feel better all day. Pressures from the day's activities don't bother you as much, and you are more pleasant to your family and your co-workers. You also have more energy, a better appetite, and a more relaxed sense about you. Plus, you never have that nagging thought in the back of your mind that you should exercise when you get home. You've already done it.

The other advantage of early morning is the sunrise. Most people never see the sunrise and its magnificent array of colors. Yet observing the sunrise can be an uplifting, awe-inspiring experience. At dawn you see unusual cloud formations on the horizon, and at times the sunlight piercing through the clouds makes them look like distant mountain ranges. There is no other time of day when you will see the clouds shaped this way.

In the winter, when you walk in the predawn morning, you can look up and see the sky filled with stars. Most of the artificial lights from houses and businesses are out, so the stars seem brighter and more abundant. Almost as wonderful as the sunrise is the moon setting. Every early morning you walk in the winter, you get to see the moon in its phases. When there is snow on the ground and the moon is in its fuller phases, the reflection from the stars and moon brings the trees and landscape into bright relief.

For early morning walks, we recommend using the buddy system. Not only does your commitment to your buddy motivate you but it is good to have a companion for safety and a sense of security, particularly in winter, when it is dark out.

In summer you often go from air-conditioned house to air-conditioned car to air-conditioned office. Early morning walks are great at this time of year because this is the coolest time of day and the temperature is quite pleasant. It's also a great time to be out in the sunshine without damaging your skin.

Getting Up Early

Whenever you want to change a habit and form a new one, you need to repeat a behavior without fail for an extended period of time. If you want to reset your body clock so that you are an early riser, you need to get up at the same hour every day for at least a month, preferably eight weeks. Once you have gotten into the habit of getting up early, you should try to keep on that schedule even on the weekends, rising within not more than an hour of your normal wake-up time. At first you will need the help of an alarm clock, but after about a year your body will reset its inner clock and you will automatically wake up at an early hour. Even if, on occasion, you go to bed really late at night, you will still be able to get up early. And, remember, you have your buddy. You are not going to let a friend sit out in the cold and dark by herself.

The process of getting up early actually starts the evening before, with going to bed early. This may seem hard to manage, especially if you have kids, but if you can remember that you and your kids will be much happier and healthier if you get a good night's sleep, it may motivate you to organize the family around an early bedtime. As an early riser, you will never have trouble sleeping at night. Your insomnia will be a distant memory. You can go to bed at 10:00 P.M., get up by 5:00 or 5:30 A.M., and still get an appropriate amount of sleep. You will find that the seven to seven and a half hours of sleep you get with this schedule will feel ample because your sleep will be much deeper thanks to your regular walking yoga practice.

When you get up at 5:00 or 6:00 A.M., you may feel sleepy around 3:00 in the afternoon. A mid-afternoon energy lull can be easily managed by going for another short walk or taking ten minutes to do some deep breathing. If you have to go out that night, take a fifteen-minute Yoga Nidra (yogic sleep) by practicing the Corpse pose (see page 88) before you leave for the evening. This will give you the lift you need to carry you through to bedtime.

Getting up early is a lot easier if you don't eat too much or too late at night. Because we use eating not just for nourishment but for pleasure and as an antidote to stress, it is hard to stop eating late into the night, or eating until your stomach hurts. One way to break this habit is to eat moderately at dinner and not eat anything sweet after dinner. Try this for at least two weeks. We find that once you have eaten dinner, you won't eat anything else unless it is sweet. Sweets are so good it is hard to eat them moderately, and you can easily consume way too much of them. Going to bed feeling stuffed on sweets makes it much harder to get up.

Some people find it impossible not to eat sweets after dinner. One reason you crave sweets so much is that your dinner is too salty. Try to eat a meal that has a balance of salt and includes sweet vegetables such as carrots, sweet potatoes, tomatoes, or zucchini. Then have a cup of hot herbal tea with a little honey in it or a small portion of cooked or fresh fruit after dinner to help satisfy your craving for a sweet.

If you can get to bed earlier, rise at the same hour every morning, and eat moderately at dinner with no sweets afterwards for at least four weeks, you will find it easy to stick to your early morning walking yoga practice.

EARLY EVENING

Evening walks help you unwind from the day, process unfinished thoughts, and transition between your day job and your other job of running a household. Much of the conflict in relationships comes from not feeling good about ourselves. When we feel tired and overworked, we tend not to take care of ourselves, and when we don't do something that helps us feel good inside and gives us energy, we tend to be less tolerant of those around us. Taking time to nurture yourself and de-stress will help you enjoy being with your family and give you the extra energy you need to manage your household.

Taking a break after work in the early evening will also help you avoid overeating and help you digest your dinner better because you use walking yoga, not a box of cookies, to relax. Since you eat more moderately and digest your food better, you will find that your sleep is much deeper and that in the morning you feel completely rested instead of sluggish and groggy. It is a wonderful feeling to wake up early and want to get out of bed instead of wanting to avoid your life and pull the blankets back over your head. In fact, evening walking yoga helps you feel so good when you wake up in the morning that you may actually consider getting up earlier than usual to do it all over again!

Practicing walking yoga in the evening also gives you a chance to watch the sun set. Walking while the sun sets is a marvelous way to end your day and take pleasure in watching light turn to dark, orange turn to purple, then to black, and to experience the blanket of quiet that descends over the earth. In the winter you can watch as the stars begin to appear in the sky and the moon makes its ascent into the heavens above. Evening walking lets you relax and exhale as the entire world prepares for sleep.

Early evening is nice for city walkers because there is a noticeable shift in the mood of people on the streets. People seem more relaxed because the day is over, more playful, sometimes singing out loud as they walk home from work, and moving just a bit more slowly than their daytime pace.

Walking Through the Seasons

Walking every day allows you to appreciate and experience the changing seasons and the life cycles of plants, flowers, trees, insects, and animals. You can follow the phases of the moon and changing times of sunrise and sunset and get a close view of blooming flowers, migrating birds, buzzing bees, falling leaves, harvest moons, frozen ponds, and the birth and death that are all part of the cycles of life. When you walk every day, you experience the whole spectrum of life outside your car, your house, and your workplace. Life seems fuller, time seems to slow down, and you feel part of a larger world and universe.

GLORIOUS SPRING

Spring is our favorite time of the year to walk. Spring reminds us of youth, rebirth, fresh starts, and new beginnings. It's wonderful to watch the season change day by day—the leaf buds emerge from their winter casings a fresh, vivid green, the first crocus pops through the ground, often before the snow has melted, and the robin hunts for worms to feed her young. The soft touch of a warm, richly scented spring breeze caresses your face and skin so gently that your whole body relaxes.

You can closely watch the blooming of all the spring flowers. Perhaps there is no more glorious sight than the emergence of the tulip, daffodil, hyacinth, forsythia, and violet after a long, cold, gray winter. Even more intoxicating is the rich scent of the lilac bush.

If you live in the country or can get to a local park, be sure to plan longer weekend hikes to watch the rushing rivers, streambeds, and lakes swollen with snowmelt and spring rains. When you walk in springtime, you can witness firsthand the rebirth of the land as the animals wake up from their winter slumber and begin to build nests, hives, holes, and dams; forage for food; and start the miraculous process of bearing young. The melody of the songbird, the raucous yet synchronous sound of spring peepers, and the deep, sonorous croak of the bullfrog are comforting reminders that spring has finally arrived.

Spring walking is a great time to meet your neighbors and find ideas for planting your gardens. People are outside in the spring getting things ready for warmer weather, replacing storm windows with screens, painting their houses, and preparing garden beds for flowers and vegetables. You can also find out a lot by walking through your neighborhood and meeting the people who live near you.

Spring is also a great time for fresh starts. If you got out of your walking yoga discipline during the winter, it is easy to start up again in the spring, because suddenly there are more hours of daylight. In spring the sun rises earlier and the days grow longer. It is easier to do your walking yoga in the morning before work because you naturally wake up with the sun. Spring walking will help to take off the extra pounds we tend to put on in winter and relieve any lingering symptoms of winter depression.

SUMPTUOUS SUMMER

The bright green colors of spring gradually mature into the dark greens of summer. When you walk in summer your senses are treated to a multitude of colors, scents, tastes, and tactile sensations. There is something quite sensuous about walking in the hot, moist, thickly scented air of summer, and you can walk mostly free from clothing, enjoying the heat on your skin and the easy movement of your body.

When you walk in summer you can teach yourself to recognize the wildlife around you. Learning to identify the trees and flowers, the birds by their calls, and the animals by their droppings gives you a good feeling. When you walk on a summer morning and know the sound of the mourning dove or recognize the lightning-quick swallow chasing the slow-moving crow from her nest, it gives more depth to your experience. You begin to know your world just a little better, helping you to feel more a part of it.

Summertime is a great time to make your walks longer and more adventurous. Daylong hikes that venture deep into the wilds, letting you explore new trails, carry a picnic lunch, and find a place to swim are really fun. You can walk to places where you can pick wild berries or discover a variety of wildflowers. In the Northeast, mountain laurel blooms for a two-week period in summer, and when you walk through forests of laurel it is like being showered with pink and white petals in a wedding procession. Hiking vacations in summer, where you spend most of your time outdoors, are a great way to get in better shape physically and spend quality time with your loved ones.

Summertime walks tend to be more playful as well. Walking before and after thunderstorms brings out the kid in you. It will inspire awe at nature's power and sheer delight in spotting rainbows. Playing in the ocean waves as you walk along a beach, especially at sunrise or sunset, is a truly sublime experience that you will never forget. Best of all, walking in the summer helps to slow time down and makes your summer seem to last a little longer.

There is no better time of year to walk in late evening than summer. You'll catch glimpses of fireflies in flight while walking to the soothing melody of the cricket's song. Warm summer nights are the perfect time to walk slowly through your neighborhood or campsite, or on your apartment rooftop, and turn your gaze toward the heavens. Stars and planets have attracted humans for thousands of years, making astronomy the oldest known science. The stars can tell you time, location, and position but, most important, stargazing ignites the imagination. In the Northern Hemisphere, you can try to spot all the major circumpolar constellations, such as the Big and Little Dippers, Draco the dragon, Cassiopeia, and Cepheus as they rotate around Polaris, the North Star. In the Southern Hemisphere, you can spot the Southern Cross, which points to the southern celestial pole, and Sirius, the brightest star in the sky.

Your walking yoga practice can mature and deepen when you keep up your practice from spring into summer. If you have been consistent with your practice, you are sure to reap the benefits of a stronger, leaner, healthier body and a more fulfilled and confident attitude.

FALL COLORS

Walking in fall, particularly in the Northeast, is like getting to see fireworks every day. The leaves of deciduous trees and plants turn from green to red, orange, yellow, and deep maroon as the hot days of August change to the cooler days of September. The trees seem to be on fire, the landscape is a riot of color, and the overall scene is so breathtaking you can't help but feel good. The cool air of fall invigorates, motivates, and activates our desire to be outside and is the perfect weather for practicing walking yoga. The temperate conditions still allow for light clothing, yet it is cool enough to accommodate the increase in body temperature generated by the walk.

Fall walking is a great way to maintain the good feelings you get from summer weather. It's hard not to feel a bit sad when you see signs of fall coming on. Childhood memories of summer's end and the dread of going back to school make the coming of fall a bittersweet experience. The end of summer for many of us represents an end to an easier, more carefree time. Walking in the fall helps make the transition quite enjoyable as you relish the feast of fall's bounty and enjoy the amazing colors.

Winter can be the hardest time to keep up your walking yoga practice, but it is surprisingly enjoyable when you persevere. When you walk in winter, more than any other time of year, you experience a real sense of accomplishment. There is something about braving eight-degree weather that gives you a feeling of being indomitable. And it's fun to tell people that you walk in winter, because they are always impressed.

When the weather turns cold and the days grow shorter, we are more susceptible to low energy and depression. We tend to sleep and eat more in winter because of the colder weather and the holidays. A recent study conducted by the University of Massachusetts found that people were more likely to feel depressed, irritable, angry, or anxious in winter than in any other season.

Walking yoga helps to counteract the winter blues. In addition to increasing the flow of endorphins in the body, a regular walking practice can be a catalyst for other more healthy activities, which will help improve your mood. It will also burn calories and reduce your cravings for comfort foods. Walking yoga in the winter also increases your exposure to sunlight, which helps to combat depression.

Winter is a time for hibernation and inward focus. Particularly in the northern climates, the world seems to be resting in deep sleep. Winter is a good time for solitude and quiet contemplation, and if you put on your warm layers and get moving with walking yoga, you will find you have many positive life benefits to consider in your reflections.

Making a Commitment to a Walking Yoga Practice

You can only make a commitment to something when the experience generated by your commitment gives you more fulfillment and satisfaction than you would have if you didn't do it. But you have to nurture your love for good things in order to have the uplifting experience of what it feels like to be whole and healthy. In other words, doing good things for yourself will feel worse in the beginning because breaking addictions is painful. You have to understand on a whole body level the negative consequences of living an unhealthy, addictive lifestyle. Only then can you make a shift in your life and replace your old ways of being with newer, healthier habits.

If you have the desire to make changes in your health and in how you deal with stress, your best success will come when you give yourself the experience of the cause and effect of your lifestyle. For example, when you drink too much, don't take painkillers to ease the effects of the hangover. Or when you eat too much, don't take Alka-Seltzer or Rolaids to ease your indigestion. You have to experience the pain and discomfort of excessive eating and drinking so that next time you consider drinking alcohol, your memory won't be of the initial high but will be of the painful hangover. Next time you consider eating foods you know you can't digest, instead of thinking of the initial pleasure you'll remember the indigestion you experienced. It may take a while to get the lesson, but eventually this experience will motivate you to change your habits.

Designing your life so that you crave things that are good for you more than you crave destructive and unhealthy habits can be approached from two directions. The first is to learn to deal with the seductive nature of the mind. For example, no matter how bad you feel after overindulging in food or alcohol, as soon as you feel even a little better you start to think about overindulging again. The mind has an ironclad relationship with addiction, remembering the high of that first sip, bite, or drag while ignoring the painful side effects. When the body needs exercise to cleanse your system of stress, the mind starts to complain just like a child resisting bedtime or a bath. The mind, like a child, is amazingly adept at arguing its case when it wants something, even if it is bad for you. Just as a skilled parent gently lures the unsuspecting child to do what's good for him or her, you need to be skillful in enticing your mind to do what you know is best for yourself. The key is nurturing your body so that taking care of yourself gives you more pleasure than not.

The second approach is literally to reset the chemistry of the body by purifying it. You don't realize how bad you feel indulging in an addiction or habit until you have stopped it for a solid period of time. When you fast from a certain habit, such as eating sugar or drinking alcohol, you begin to feel so good that you can't imagine why you didn't quit sooner. Two things motivate us to quit bad habits. The first is pain and the second pleasure.

Most of us can relate to the experience, especially when we hit our forties, of consuming one or two drinks at a weekend party and waking up the next day with a bad hangover. We end up lying around all day and wasting one of our precious days off because we have no energy. Pretty soon we quit drinking entirely because the momentary high isn't worth feeling bad the next day. Alcohol has a more extreme and detrimental affect on the body, but most habits, such as sugar and caffeine consumption, suppress the body's energy and its natural urges for healthy living. The more sensitive you become, the less you'll be able to tolerate things that are bad for you and the more you'll enjoy those habits that give you energy.

The other motivator for quitting bad habits is the pleasurable feeling you get when you do good things for yourself. The more you eat right and exercise, the better you feel, and the better you feel, the more you crave doing good things for yourself. We do things habitually because of the pleasure we get from them. Some habits, while giving you pleasure initially, end up being more painful than not. The only way to give up pleasures that are bad for you is to replace them with pleasures that sustain you. You are human, and human beings love pleasure and resist pain. It is our nature. So design your lifestyle in such a way that it gives you lots of pleasure. Just replace pleasure that is harmful to you with pleasure that is good for you, and do this in a graduated way.

You don't need to give up your comfort foods and recreational drugs all at once. Simply moderate your intake so that it doesn't interfere with starting a walking yoga practice. With a regular practice, including the postures, breathing exercises, and walking, you will start to feel less dependent on these other stimulants and you will become more sensitive to their negative side effects. Bad habits will begin to drop away automatically, and you will crave the experience you get from your walking yoga practice. You can get that high you are seeking from food and recreational drugs in a more natural way, and you won't suffer the mood swings caused by sugar, alcohol, and marijuana.

Finally, nothing derails a regular practice more than self-judgment and unrealistic expectation. You have to consider your life circumstances when determining how much time you should practice every day. If you are a mother with young kids and a full-time job, your practice will look much different from that of someone with grown kids or no kids. Most important is to do something that nurtures you every day. Getting a good night's sleep and eating well are often the first places to start nurturing yourself.

Recommendations for Making Walking Yoga a Lifelong Practice

Our students always ask us how much time they should spend practicing. Here are some recommendations that you can tailor to your own circumstances.

- Commit to a solid period of time in which you will practice yoga and/or walking every day. The most important thing is to get started. You are aiming for a daily practice of yoga and walking of 45 minutes to an hour; listen to your own instincts about how to get there. We recommend committing to a daily practice for four weeks when you are beginning. In this way you will break any bad habits and replace them with the new habit of feeling good with yoga and walking. Good habits multiply. The more good things you do for yourself, the more good things you want to do. Your body will actually start to crave the experience of stretching and exercise.

- During the initial four-week period, try to spend at least 30 minutes walking and 30 minutes doing hatha yoga every day. Taking a yoga class once a week is a good idea for beginners. On weekends increase your walking to an hour if possible.

- If you can't afford the time, start with 15 minutes per day of any form of walking yoga. If nothing else, practice Yoga Nidra (Corpse pose, see page 88) and Ujjayi breathing (see page 101) before you go to sleep.

- Find a favorite street or path where you feel safe to walk, and find a buddy to accompany and support you. If you have a baby, put the baby in a stroller and head out for your walking yoga session.

- Pick a favorite time to walk every day. Consistency helps regularity.

- Periodically do a more intensive practice by taking a retreat either by yourself or with a group. In-depth study and concentrated practice, particularly with a group, help to keep you motivated and inspired.

- Let failure teach you, not discourage you. When you stop practicing, notice how you feel. At some point you will come back to your routine. Judging yourself drains energy more often than it motivates. No matter how busy you are, you can always practice Ujjayi breathing, and that will eventually lead you back to your practice.

If you take away anything from this book, remember that you can access the power of walking yoga when you are fully present in your practice. Being fully present in the moment allows you to tune in to your body's natural intelligence and approach your life with skillfulness and equilibrium. When you become creative at inspiring the mind and effective in reducing addictive habits that weaken the body, you can reliably trust your instincts for how and when to practice walking yoga. Be gentle, nurture yourself, and have fun exploring your world on foot.

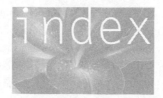

index

Page numbers of illustrations appear in italics.

conscious breathing and walking,
115–16
crosslateral motion and, 105
of motion, 104
patterns of movement, poor
posture and, 111
practicing, Yoga Mudra, 42–43
Shiva, 136
Shoulders
Downward Dog, 69–70, 69
Forearm Stretch, 58–59, 58
Shoulder Stand, thyroid, pineal
glands and, 13
Warrior, 74–76, 75, 76
Yoga Mudra, 83–85, 83, 84
Sinus, clearing, Kapalabhati
breathing and, 102–3
Skeletal system, 10–11
stiffness and, 38–39
Skillful action, 8, 145
as integration of inertia and
growth, 8
walking yoga and, 16
yoga and mastery of the postures,
8, 29
Smoking, quitting, Ujjayi breathing
and, 101–2
Solar plexus, 107, 125–26. *See also*
Chakras, third
Spine, 10–11, 12
Cobra pose, 80–82, 81
Forward Bend, 85, 86, 87–88
Knee Down Twist, 54–56, 55
intervertebral disks, 10
Locust pose, 79–80, 80
Supine Leg Stretch, 49, 50,
51–52

Spirituality
breathing and, 13
contemplative walking and,
155–56
dynamic practice, various
religions, 6
sensitivity to experiences of the
body and, 36
walking yoga and, 5, 16
Spring Hill Music, 136–37
Standing Back Bend, 61–62, 62
Standing Forward Bend, 62–63, 63
Standing postures, 74–79
Tree pose, 77–79, 78
Warrior, 74–76, 75, 76
Stress
adrenaline, cortisol release and,
14
cause of illness and disease, 14
Child pose for lower back
tension, 56–58, 57
conscious breathing and walking
to reduce, 116
contemplative walking for, 156
exercise to reduce, 26–27
flight or fight response, 14
Forearm Stretch for tension in
arms and shoulders, 58–59, 58
Neck Roll for releasing tension in
neck and shoulders, 45
soothing posture, Downward
Dog, 69–70, 69
walking for reducing, 14, 15, 26
Warrior for tension in neck and
shoulders, 74–76, 75, 76
yoga for reducing or countering,
12, 26, 39